# I WANT TO LIVE
## Using
# Essiac

*For anyone who is fighting cancer, helping others
who have cancer, or trying to prevent cancer.
The truth about Essiac.*

CAROLINE DEHARDE BENNETT

ISBN:      1480164844

ISBN 13:   9781480164840

Library of Congress Control Number: 2012920164
CreateSpace Independent Publishing Platform
North Charleston, South Carolina

# Description

Why are you reading this book? Does someone you know have cancer? Do you have cancer? Are you going to be taking care of someone who has cancer? Or, perhaps you want to prevent your family members and yourself from ever getting cancer. If these are any of the reasons for reading this book, you are making the best decision of your life.

**Are we winning the battle against cancer?** Today, in the United States and Canada, the three main treatments for dealing with cancer are surgery, chemotherapy, and radiation. For a few kinds of cancer, such as skin cancer, surgery can save someone's life. The dreaded diseases of childhood cancers are uniquely susceptible to chemotherapy and radiation. However, for everyone else, chemotherapy and radiation will only slow down the cancer's progression and leave patients fighting all the damage done to their immune systems.

When someone hears that she has cancer, does she feel secure, safe, or petrified? It is because of these feelings of apprehension that I sought out a truly helpful therapy that would strengthen the immune system and thus possibly prevent cancer. Is this therapy new? No, it has been around since the 1920s. Before then, it was used by the Ojibwa (Chippewa Indians) as a cancer cure. The cancer therapy is called Essiac, and it was discovered by Rene Caisse, RN.

Have you ever heard of Essiac? When someone tries to find out about Essiac online, he might find one site on cancer therapies hosted by Quackwatch, which states that Essiac has no antitumor activity. This is totally untrue.

Several books have been written on Essiac, but I have pulled together research and proof that has not been written about before. I will offer proof that Essiac, an alternative cancer approach, does alter and stop cancer. There is evidence that Essiac really does work when it is used as it is supposed to be. Besides having found many research projects that tell how Essiac and its component herbs have antitumor activity, I have also discovered that in 1996, China's department of health declared the Essiac formula a Class A medicine—one that deals with life-threatening diseases—and since then, it has been used to treat cancer in China. Quite notably, it has demonstrated a clear ability to inhibit the growth of tumors.

The work that I have gathered goes into everything regarding Essiac, including the history of Essiac's initial use by Rene M. Caisse RN, who spent fifty years of her life treating people with cancer.

Essiac is touted by Sir Frederick Banting (the discoverer of insulin), Dr. Emma M. Carson (recipient of awards from Presidents Roosevelt and Wilson), and Dr. Charles Brusch (personal physician to President John F. Kennedy). But most importantly, there is proof today that after ninety years of using it, even without standard protocol, direct evidence shows that Essiac does work.

This books shows that the natural herbs that comprise Essiac, which were originally offered by the Ojibwa Indians, do have a preventative and/or healing effect on cancer.

*May the words of an Ojibwa Medicine Man remain with us.*

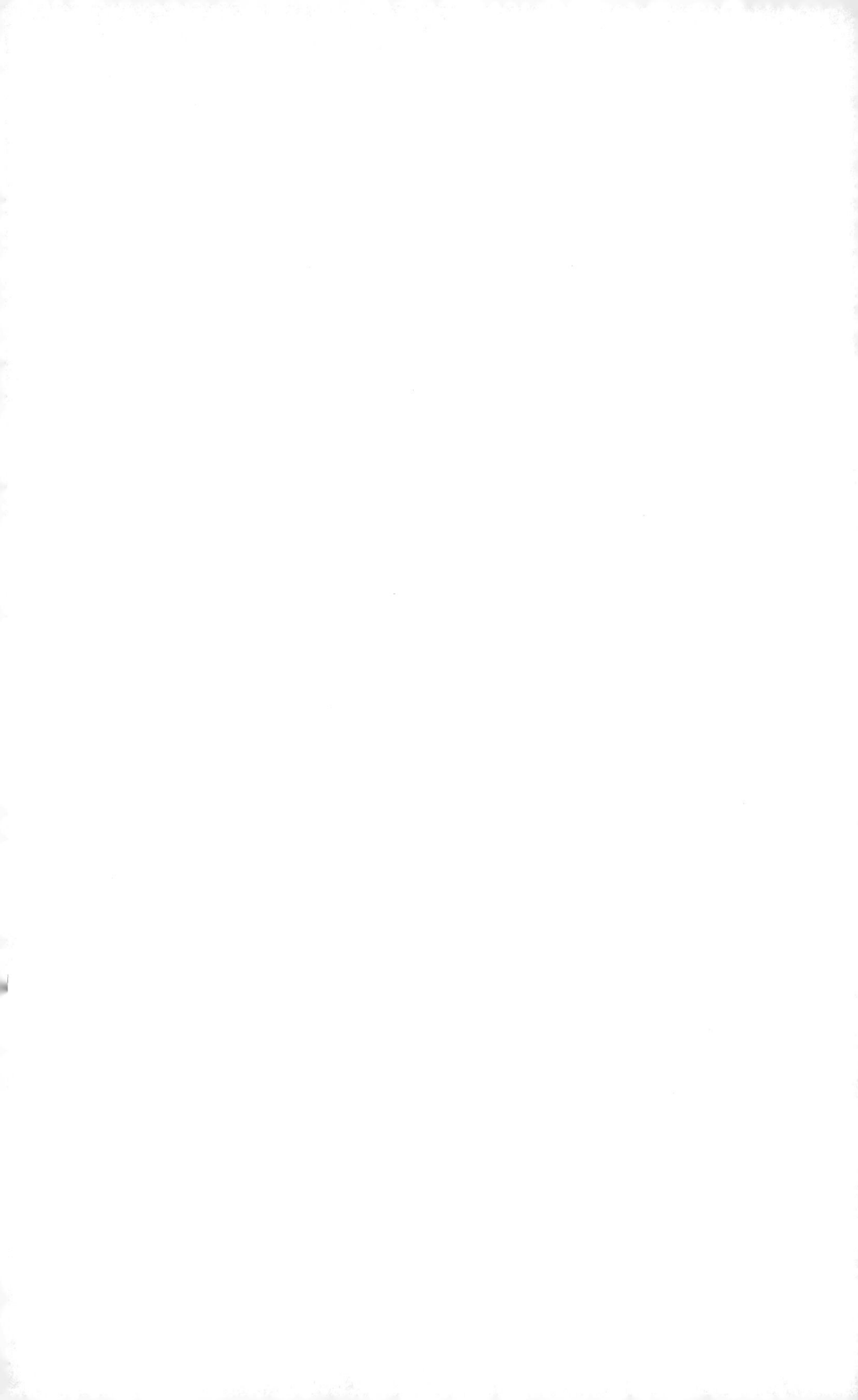

# Table of Contents

# Introduction

Essiac, an herbal remedy used as an alternative cancer therapy, has an impressive anecdotal history of success in the United States and Canada, and newer clinical data warrants further research for use in complementary/ conventional cancer treatment. The objective of this book is threefold. The first goal is to increase awareness of the alternative cancer treatment called Essiac. The second is to provide evidence that its history warrants that it be reliably and thoroughly investigated clinically in the United States and Canada. Most importantly, the third goal is to provide information to those who suffer from cancer, to those who wish to prevent cancer, and to those who provide treatment and care for individuals afflicted with the disease.

This material includes a complete history of Essiac and its creator, Rene Caisse RN. She had the unwavering quest to help as many cancer sufferers as possible during her long life. This book provides a detailed discussion of Essiac's component herbs, and its safety and efficacy is compared and contrasted to conventional cancer therapies. International use and availability of Essiac to cancer patients is covered. Further, the prevalence of and reasons for using complementary/alternative medicine (CAM) are explored. Finally, the implications of Essiac use and other CAM modalities to the medical field today will be discussed. These objectives and methods yield substantial support for the need for further clinical investigation of Essiac in the United States and Canada.

# HISTORY OF ESSIAC AND RENE CAISSE

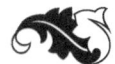

It is vital that everyone who reads this book knows and understands the true nature and distinguishing characteristics of Rene Caisse. Therefore, we will start with her life and everything that was important to her.

Essiac (pronounced ess-E-ack) is the name given to the herbal cancer remedy created by a Canadian nurse named Rene Caisse early in the twentieth century. She came up with the name for her remedy by reversing the letters of her surname.

Rene Caisse was born on August 11, 1888, in Bracebridge, Ontario. She was one of seventeen children born to Friselda and Joseph Caisse. Friselda was a seamstress by trade, and Joseph, a barber. Together they raised Rene and her ten surviving siblings in a loving, but strict, Roman Catholic tradition.

Rene attended Catholic elementary school and gradu-
ated from continuation school in 1904. She worked briefly
in Toronto in 1907, and in 1908, she worked one summer as
a stewardess on a luxury steamboat vessel on the Muskoka
Lakes. It was in 1909 that Rene would embark on her jour-
ney to fulfill her dreams of becoming a nurse and helping
"suffering humanity." At age twenty-one, she left her hometown and headed to Greenwich, Connecticut, to study
nursing at a private hospital under the tutelage of Dr. Fritz
Carlton Hyde and his wife, who was also a physician. A year
later, Rene returned to Bracebridge as a graduate nurse, and
she worked as a private duty nurse in people's homes until
1912.

During the time that Rene was in Greenwich studying,
a typhoid fever epidemic broke out in northern Ontario.
The Red Cross hospitals were in dire need, and they advertised for nurses to aid the sick and suffering. Rene made
the decision to head north during one of the coldest win-
ters in history to take a position with the Red Cross for fifty
dollars a month plus free room and board. She divided her
time between rather primitive outpost hospitals and a more
modern hospital in Cobalt. Many of her patients were silver
miners, prospectors, and their families. Between the years
1913 and 1914, the Sisters of Providence bought the Cobalt
hospital and built a larger one in nearby Haileybury. At this
location, they were better equipped to treat the typhoid
patients. During this time, Rene took additional courses and
advanced to head nurse.

In 1915, at the age of twenty-seven, Rene decided to leave
northern Ontario as she was emotionally drained from her
work with the sick and dying. Further, she was still single

and missed her family. Rene would first live with her sister, Louise, and her husband, Otto, in Alberta, and then in Manitoba. However, following the death of her father (aged sixty-one) in 1916, she returned to live with her mother in Toronto.

While in Toronto, she continued nursing, and took classes six hours per week to help her advance toward her RN designation. Her nursing experience involved assisting in several doctors' offices. It was at this time that she first worked with Dr. Robert O. Fisher. She and Dr. Fisher would go on to be colleagues for years.

It was sometime during Rene's early years of nursing that she learned of an herbal cancer remedy. Some sources cite 1922 as the year of discovery, but this is not certain. Rene often spoke of first hearing about the remedy for cancer while working up north, which would have been earlier than 1922. One of Rene's patients was an elderly Englishwoman. While one of the woman's nurses was bathing her, Rene noticed that the woman's breast was a mass of scar tissue. Rene questioned the Englishwoman and recorded the account of their discussion:

> "I came out of England nearly thirty years ago," she told me. "I joined my husband, who was prospecting in the wilds of Northern Ontario. My right breast became sore and swollen, and very painful. My husband brought me to Toronto, and the doctors told me I had advanced cancer and my breast must be removed at once. Before we left camp, a very old Indian medicine man had told me I had cancer, but he could cure it. I decided I'd just as soon try his remedy as to have my breast removed. One of my friends had died from breast surgery. Besides, we had no money."

She and her husband returned to the mining camp, and the old Indian showed her certain herbs growing in the area, told her to make tea from these herbs, and to drink it every day. She was nearly eighty years old when I saw her, and there had been no recurrence of cancer. I was much interested, and wrote down the names of the herbs she had used. I knew that doctors threw up their hands when cancer was discovered in a patient; it was the same as a death sentence, just about. I decided that if I should ever develop cancer, I would use this herb tea.

About a year later, I was visiting an aged retired doctor whom I knew well. We were walking slowly about his garden when he took his cane and lifted a weed. "Nurse Caisse," he told me, "if people would use this weed, there would be little or no cancer in the world." He told me the name of the plant. It was one of the herbs my patient had named as an ingredient of the Indian medicine man's tea! (Caisse 1966, 1-2)

It is generally speculated that the medicine man was an Ojibwa (Chippewa) Indian. That tribe inhabited the Lake Country in Canada during the time the Englishwoman described. An Ojibwa medicine man would have been a member of the Grand Medicine society called the Midewiwin, and he would have been trained for four to eight years. "It has been said that the [Ojibwa] tribes around the Great Lakes were familiar with as many as four hundred plants for treating illness" (Olson 1998, 40).

Although these two interchanges were most interesting to Rene, little did she know at the time that they would greatly affect the remainder of her life. "These events inadvertently set the course of her working life, spanning almost the next five decades, thrusting her into a medical-legal-political controversy that stretched across the province and into the United States" (Ivey 2004, 55).

Rene tucked away the herbal formula for future use, and the future came quite quickly. In 1924, Rene's aunt, Mireza Potvin, was operated on in a Brockville hospital, where a biopsy was performed. "She was diagnosed by two prominent doctors as having terminal cancer of the stomach, with liver involvement, and was given six months or less to live. Apparently, the whole stomach was so corrugated with the disease that they simply closed up the wound and left her to die" (Caisse 1966, 2). Mireza was discharged to be cared for until her death in the home of her sister, Friselda (Rene's mother), under the care of Dr. R. O. Fisher.

It was at this time that Rene told Dr. Fisher of the herbal tea, and asked that she might treat her aunt with it. Since there was no other medical intervention that could save the woman's life, Dr. Fisher readily agreed. Rene gathered the herbs, brewed the tea, and administered it daily to her aunt. After about two months, her condition improved remarkably, so much so that she could return to her own home. She continued to improve and went on to live an additional twenty-one years.

Dr. Fisher was so impressed with Mireza's recovery that he asked Rene to make the tea for some of his other cancer patients who were hopeless. Word of Miss Caisse's herbal tea began to spread, and soon other doctors in the area began to show an interest in the herbal remedy for their hopeless cases. Around this time, Rene Caisse named the tea Essiac, which is her last name spelled backward.

Dr. Fisher helped her to set up a makeshift lab, in which they tested the tea on mice that had been inoculated with cancer cells. By experimenting with the different component herbs in the tea during her mice experiments, Rene was able to isolate which of the herbs was responsible for shrinking tumors. She concluded that one herb inhibited the tumors, while the others acted to strengthen the system and purify the blood. With this information, Dr. Fisher proposed that they remove the protein content of the tea and administer it to patients by injection, in addition to administering the tea orally. According to an Essiac historian, Dr. Gary L. Glum, Rene described the first injection she and Dr. Fisher administered to one of his patients from New York, who suffered from advanced cancer of the tongue and throat:

> Dr. Fisher wanted me to inject Essiac into the tongue. Well, I was nearly scared to death. And there was a violent reaction. The patient developed a severe chill; his tongue swelled so badly the doctor had to press it down with a spatula to let him breathe. That lasted about twenty minutes. Then the swelling went down, the chill subsided, and the patient was all right. The cancer stopped growing, the patient went home, and lived quite comfortably for almost four years. (Glum 1988, 18)

Rene concluded that she must learn a great deal more about Essiac before she would continue to inject patients with it. She did note, however, that all of the mice that were administered an injection, in addition to the oral preparation, demonstrated favorable results more quickly than those who were given the tea alone.

Rene continued to brew her Essiac tea for terminal cancer cases brought to her by Dr. Fisher and other nearby doctors. Two of these patients' stories are recorded in numerous publications. The first was a middle-aged Type I diabetic woman with cancer of the bowel. The doctor discontinued her insulin, so as not to interfere with the Essiac. The tea was then administered. At first, the tumor enlarged, almost obstructing the bowel, but gradually, it softened and shrank until it was all gone. The patient was treated for six months, and after that time, she had no recurrence of cancer or of diabetes.

The second patient was brought to Rene on the brink of death. He was an eighty-year-old man with huge hemorrhaging malignancies about his face and chin. Rene began treatments immediately. The hemorrhaging stopped within twenty-four hours, and after several days of treatment, the growths began to shrink. This is substantiated with photography. The man's life was prolonged comfortably for five more months, at which time he died of pneumonia.

For nearly two years, Rene continued her research with Essiac and administered it to patients referred to her by doctors. By all accounts, Essiac was improving the quality of life for many people, easing their pain, extending their lives, and causing their cancers to go into remission. Rene believed firmly that Essiac was the best cancer therapy currently available. She only wished that she could help people earlier in their diagnosis; she felt certain that her results would be even more remarkable if her patients did not seek relief having already been so badly damaged by cancer and the ensuing radium treatments.

Because they were so impressed with the remissions they had observed, eight doctors familiar with Miss Caisse's work were compelled to write and send a petition to the Canadian Health Department in October of 1926. They felt that she should be given the opportunity to research her therapy further. In their words:

> We, the undersigned, believe the treatment for cancer by Nurse R. M. Caisse can do no harm and that it relieves pain, will reduce the enlargement, and prolong life in hopeless cases.
>
> To the best of our knowledge, she has not been given a case to treat until everything in medical and surgical science has been tried without effect, and even then, she was able to show remarkably beneficial results on those cases at the late stage.
>
> We would be interested to see her given an opportunity to prove her work in a large way. To the best of our knowledge, she has treated all cases free of charge and has been carrying on this work over the period of the past two years. (Ivey 2004, 61-62)

The petition was signed by the eight physicians, dispatched, and almost immediately responded to by the government.

Despite the doctors' good intentions, and Rene's naïve belief that recognition of her therapy and research was imminent, a far different scenario was set into motion. The Department of Health and Welfare authorized two doctors to investigate Rene Caisse and her remedy. They appeared at her doorstep unannounced and with official papers in hand to have her arrested, should they see fit, for practicing medicine without a license. Rene was able to avoid arrest by explaining that she was treating only patients who had written prescriptions from their doctors, which she produced for the investigators. She also stated that she did not charge anyone for treatments. Her intelligent, thoughtful reply helped her to avoid arrest, and she was allowed to continue her work.

One of the doctors sent to investigate Nurse Caisse's work was Dr. W.C. Arnold. He was so impressed with the work she was doing that he offered her the use of the Christie Street Hospital laboratory. She would be allowed to perform tests on mice under the supervision of two staff doctors. Rene said during later interviews, "Those mice were inoculated with Rous Sarcoma. I kept them alive for fifty-two days—which was longer than anyone else had been able to do" (Glum 1988, 21). In a later experiment, under the supervision of two other doctors, the mice were kept alive with Essiac treatments for seventy-two days, an unbelievable feat.

In 1929, Rene Caisse would first meet Dr. Frederick Banting, of the Banting Institute, at the University of Toronto. Dr. Banting is the co-discoverer of insulin, which is used in the treatment of diabetes. He had heard of the diabetic patient treated by Rene who no longer needed insulin after her Essiac treatments for cancer. He had speculated that some component of the preparation had stimulated the patient's pancreas to produce insulin again. Most interested in her work, he familiarized himself with her case studies and pictures taken of patients before and after treatment. He gave important words to Rene: "Miss Caisse, I will not say you have a cure for cancer, but you have more evidence of a beneficial treatment for cancer than anyone in the world" (Olson 1998, 12).

Dr. Banting encouraged Nurse Caisse to continue her research at the University of Toronto. She seriously considered this, but ultimately declined when she learned that she would have to disclose the Essiac formula. She still had shared it with no one. She feared that it would be exploited, misused, or that she would not be credited for her research. Since her initial encounter with the Department of Health and Welfare, Rene had felt the undercurrents of persecution. She was grateful for the doctors who openly supported her work, but was very suspicious of the medical establishment. Dr. Banting supported her decision, and said he would help her if she ever changed her mind in the future.

Later that year, Rene decided to give up her professional nursing job and devote her time entirely to Essiac research and her cancer patients. She returned to Bracebridge, Ontario, where she treated an average of thirty cancer patients each day out of her apartment. She was forced to move to another apartment in the same building when neighbors complained about the constant parade of cars and people going in for treatment. This was a time of financial hardship for Rene and her fellow Canadians. It was during the Depression and unemployment was at thirty-two percent. Rene no longer had regular income, but she made due with donations from her patients. These were often in the form of food and household items.

In 1930, an agent of the Canadian College of Physicians and Surgeons showed up at Rene's apartment. He was there to issue a warrant for her arrest. The charge was practicing medicine without a license from her apartment. She again avoided arrest by proving that she was charging no fees and that she was only administering treatment to patients who had a prescription from a doctor.

Two years later, as word of Nurse Caisse's success continued to spread, many stories about her appeared in the press. A 1932 headline in the *Toronto Star* proclaimed, "Bracebridge Girl Makes Notable Discovery Against Cancer." The notoriety resulted in a threat of arrest and imprisonment, again for practicing medicine without a license. This time Rene countered, and she requested a hearing with the Minister of Health, Dr. John R. Robb. She was granted an audience, and she took along five supportive doctors and a dozen of her patients. Again, she was able to avoid prosecution, and Dr. Robb said she could continue "for now" as long as she didn't charge for her services or treat anyone not referred by a doctor.

By this point, Rene Caisse was under great stress. She was forty-four years of age and quite overweight. She worked long days administering her treatment to the never-ending line of cancer patients that were sent to her. She spent her evenings until the wee hours cooking up Essiac tea. Her determination and stamina were remarkable under the mounting political pressure.

But while Rene experienced antagonism from the establishment, she enjoyed adulation from the public. Her hometown of Bracebridge proudly embraced her and her work. The Bracebridge town council unanimously voted to donate a deserted building, formerly known as the Bracebridge Inn, for Miss Caisse to use as a treatment center. She rented the building for one dollar a month, which included utilities and a janitor. The Rene M. Caisse Cancer Clinic had five treatment rooms, a reception area, an office, and a dispensary. For the next eight years, Rene would treat thousands of patients sent to her by doctors with the Essiac formula. Most of these people were gravely ill by the time they made it to her clinic.

In 1935, Rene's mother became very ill. She was diagnosed with advanced liver cancer. Every doctor, including an internationally renowned physician named Roscoe Graham, told Rene that her mother had only days to live. Rene never told her mother that she had cancer and immediately administered Essiac, telling Friselda that it was a tonic the doctor had ordered. She gave it to her for ten consecutive days and then gradually reduced the dosage. Her mother made a complete recovery and went on to live another eighteen years. Friselda finally passed away of heart failure at age ninety.

Rene's work with cancer patients continued to garner attention and support. In 1936, feeling public pressure, the Minister of Health, Dr. James Faulkner, promised to arrange for Rene to meet again with Sir Frederick Banting (of insulin fame), and discuss her cancer research. During their meeting, Dr. Banting proposed that Rene do research on mice inoculated with mouse sarcoma and chickens inoculated with Rous sarcoma in his lab at the University of Toronto. Although Rene thought his offer was kind, she felt compelled to refuse it. Dr. Banting had made it clear that she would have to give up her clinic work. Her patients were terrified at the prospect of her leaving them, and Rene had already done research on mice. She appreciated Dr. Banting's willingness to work with her, but said she could not allow people to die in the meantime.

Later in 1936, the Canadian authorities received two more petitions, both signed by prominent physicians, urging further study of Essiac. One of these petitions conveys the sense of urgency that nine doctors felt about the benefit of Essiac, and the fear that the United States would soon act to claim the discovery if Canada continued to ignore and/ or antagonize Nurse Caisse's work. The petition sent to the Prime Minister, Minister of Health, and Attorney-General of Ontario on December 23, 1936, follows:

1. That whereas Cancer is considered the greatest scourge of humanity.
2. Whereas Miss Rene M. Caisse of Bracebridge has discovered "ESSIAC," a treatment which has proven to be a complete control, if not cure for Cancer.
3. Whereas patients treated with "ESSIAC" several years ago are still living and well.
4. Whereas Miss Caisse has pathological proof of the effectiveness of "ESSIAC," her treatment for Cancer.
5. That we as physicians and doctors of the Medical Profession recognize the importance of this treatment and are in favour of keeping it in Canada.
6. And whereas Miss Caisse is demonstrating this treatment before American University doctors, which will inevitably take her out of Canada permanently if action is not taken to keep her here.

Therefore be it resolved that we, the undersigned, do strongly urge that the Honourable, the Minister of Health take immediate action to make this treatment available for cancer sufferers, and keep it a Canadian discovery. (Ivey 2004, 106)

This petition was signed by Dr. Wm. Oaks (Rosseau), Dr. M.S. Wittick (Burks Falls), Dr. W. Dillane (Powassan), Dr. E. J. Ellis (Bracebridge), Dr. F. Shannon (Churchill),

Dr. B. l. Guyatt (Toronto), Dr. J. M. Greig, (Bracebridge), Dr. R. O. Fisher (Toronto), and Dr. J. A. McInnis (Timmins). There was no response given to either petition.

As the Canadian doctors feared, Nurse Caisse did indeed begin working with Americans. She agreed to try her treatments at Northwestern University in Chicago on tumor patients. What began with good intentions did not go as hoped. The course that Rene had laid out for herself was far too ambitious. For three winter months in 1937, she made the arduous trip across the border every other week to administer her treatment in Chicago.

On the return trip, she would stop in Toronto to treat patients and then return to Bracebridge to treat more patients. She was treating three groups of terminal cancer patients but neglecting her own health. The trips were a financial, as well as a physical, drain on her. Further, she felt that she had little control over the Chicago trials, and that she was not kept abreast of what was happening in her absence. Finally, Rene's own health deteriorated so badly that her doctors ordered that she take complete rest for two to three months for heart and nervous strain. She was cared for in the home of her sister.

Rene felt very bad about being unable to continue the Chicago trials and having to abandon the test patients, as most did not fare well without continued treatment. The ones who had been helped the most implored her, by letter, to continue, but she could not.

Later, Nurse Caisse was even offered a clinic at Passavant Hospital in Chicago. Also, a cancer specialist in Rochester, New York, named Dr. Richard Leonardo, who became quite interested in her work, offered to have her come and work with him as well. Rene declined both offers because she was reluctant to share the Essiac formula. She also had decided that she was most obligated to her Canadian patients, and she wanted to return to working with them.

In 1937, a respected cancer specialist and world traveler from Los Angeles named Dr. Emma M. Carson made the decision to travel to Bracebridge and visit Nurse Caisse's cancer clinic. Dr. Carson was the recipient of several awards by the Roosevelt and Wilson administrations. Word of Rene's work was circulating throughout medical circles in the United States, and Dr. Carson had heard of her from colleagues in Chicago. Here is an excerpt from the review she prepared after her visit:

> I was firmly resolved that my investigation be based on unprejudiced judgment. The vast majority of Miss Caisses's patients were brought to her after surgery, radiation, x-rays, emplastrums, etc. had failed to be helpful, and the patients were pronounced incurable or hopeless cases. The progress obtainable and the actual results from Essiac treatments, and the rapidity of repair were absolutely marvelous, and must have been seen to be believed.
>
> My skepticism neither yielded nor became subdued by the hopes and faith so definitely expressed by the patients and their friends. As I reviewed, compared, and summarized my data, records, case histories, etc., I realized that skepticism had deserted me. When I arrived, I contemplated remaining twelve hours—I remained twenty-four days. I examined results obtained on four hundred patients. (Olsen 1998, 14-15)

Premier Mitchell Hepburn had openly praised Nurse Caisse for her work during his bid for election. He campaigned on the promise to see that she be allowed to continue her humanitarian work unhindered and without persecution. (Rene always maintained that Mr. Hepburn had assured her that he would do all in his power to enact legislation that would permit her to practice with a medical license.)

In 1938, the number of Rene's supporters continued to swell. They wanted to put an end to her persecution and constant threat of imprisonment. They decided to work to introduce a bill to Parliament that would authorize Nurse Caisse to practice the treatment of cancer and conditions resulting from cancer—in effect, to have her declared a medical doctor in the Province of Ontario. The proposed bill was backed by a petition signed by fifty-five thousand citizens. Despite the gargantuan effort, the bill failed to pass by three votes. The public was outraged and threatened political retribution in upcoming elections. There were many accusations of collusion by a Cancer Commission, still in its infancy, and the Canadian Medical Association.

At the same time, Harold Kirby, the new Minister of Health, introduced the Kirby Bill. The bill would require investigation of unorthodox cancer treatments, for the protection of the public. Although the bill would require the investigation of all unorthodox cancer treatments, it was no secret that Essiac was the primary target of this investigation. Under the proposed bill, Rene would be required to present evidence to a committee of doctors on the benefits of Essiac. If they deemed her evidence conclusive, Essiac would then be legalized. There was one caveat, however;

the formula for Essiac needed to be turned over to the commission. The bill stipulated that if Rene were to refuse, but continue to treat patients, she would be subject to fines and imprisonment. The Kirby Bill did require that commission members keep the formula confidential; although, no punitive provisions were incorporated into the legislation should the formula be accidentally divulged. The Bill was tabled in March of 1938, but reintroduced and passed in June of that year. Rene expressed her outrage:

> The people of Ontario will be paying a group of men to develop something that was developed and discovered fifteen years ago. I have developed and proven a cure right here in Bracebridge, and I am running a clinic where hundreds of cancer sufferers are being treated and helped.
>
> Why then should I be asked to give my formula over to a group of doctors who never did anything to earn it? If the Ontario legislature can pass a law to put me in jail for six months for helping suffering people, I will close my clinic and go to the United States. I shall not buck such opposition. (Thomas 1993, 25)

On June 1, 1938, Rene closed the clinic under fear of prosecution. Her patients tearfully implored her to remain open, and the public continued to deluge the government with letters of support and outrage. During the clinic closure, many of Rene's patients who had been in remission took a turn for the worse, and many of her sicker patients died. It was a heartbreaking situation for Rene.

It was during this time that Rene quietly married a good friend, a widower named Charles McGaughey. He was a respected barrister from North Bay, which was a two-hour train ride from Bracebridge. Rene was now fifty years old. She took her husband's surname, but remained Rene Caisse professionally.

On August 5, 1938, Rene relented and reopened the clinic. She could no longer ignore people's suffering. Further, it was ascertained by her husband and government officials that she could not be prosecuted before the convening of the Cancer Commission. However, things were not the same. She still had not disclosed the formula to anyone, but the number of patients coming to her with prescriptions from their doctors had noticeably declined. Some of the doctors who had been sending patients to Rene were now reluctant to do so because of the growing controversy. Patients told Rene that their doctors were under huge pressure from their peers, and that their practices would be threatened should they still work with her.

During the last months of 1938, Rene continued to treat cancer patients, all the while fending off the Cancer Commission that was getting underway. She still refused to turn over the formula for Essiac if they were unwilling to acknowledge the proof of its effectiveness as evidenced by her years of work and good results. They refused to accept her evidence without knowing the formula and testing it themselves.

In March of 1939, The Cancer Commission finally convened at the Royal Oak Hotel in Toronto. Rene Caisse would formally present her cases through written record and through the personal testimonies of her patients. She arrived at the hearing with so many supporters that they filled a ballroom. Among these supporters were three hundred eighty-seven patients, all of who were ready to testify before the Commission. The Commission allowed only forty-nine of Rene's patients to tell their stories, in the interest of expediency.

These forty-nine patients would all describe the debilitating effects of their cancer, and many described their radium burns from treatment. All told of their doctors' diagnoses and of being given only a short time to live. They had all ended up on the clinic's doorstep because of their dire situations. The patients' stories were emotional and powerful. Each person described how the Essiac treatments had helped him or her to regain health. All the patients had been declared hopeless by their doctors, but they now described the recoveries: some partial, some continuing, and many remarkably complete. The words miracle and miraculous were used often during the testimony.

Rene felt that the Commission could not deny the validity of her treatment after hearing this overwhelming evidence. But to her surprise, she was again asked at this point to relinquish her formula for further testing. She refused again, in disbelief, and that was the end of the proceedings for that day.

Three weeks later, the doctors were to testify before the Cancer Commission. There were several documents submitted signed by doctors who said that their patients had not benefited from Essiac and had subsequently died. These were all read before the Commission and Rene Caisse. The Commissioner concluded, from these testimonies, that Rene was not able to cure an advanced stage of cancer.

In her defense, Rene countered that no one could have cured some of the patients who had come to her. Their organs had already been destroyed, and she could not rebuild bodies. She said in those cases, she was happy that her treatments were at least able to help them live out their final days more comfortably.

The Commissioner then pointed out that some of the cures that Rene was crediting to Essiac might really have been the result of the radium treatments the patients had received prior to being treated at her cancer clinic. Rene responded, "In other words, if the patient lives, you take the credit for radium, but if the patient dies, radium has nothing to do with it" (Glum 1988, 85).

What is very important is that the doctors' reports did admit that many patients had experienced relief from pain, and there were no reports of Essiac causing harm, but the body of the doctors' testimony was a campaign to discredit Rene Caisse and Essiac. Rene was devastated by this betrayal and completely caught off guard by the venom she endured. After all, she had only taken cases that had been given up as hopeless by the medical establishment, and although Rene was not given the opportunity to respond to each of the doctors' testimonies during this hearing, she would later respond to each one in writing, but to no avail.

The hearing was ended with one more request that Rene turn over the formula for Essiac. Rene responded, "I want to know that suffering humanity will benefit by it. When I can be given that assurance, I am willing to disclose my formula, but I have got to know that it is going to get to suffering humanity" (Glum 1988, 86). The Commission refused to admit the merit of Essiac based on testimony alone, so again, Rene Caisse denied them the formula. Why did the

Cancer Commission, which saw no worth in Essiac, ask for the formula three times?

The Cancer Commission would take months to write their report. During this time, Rene lived through the heartbreak of having to turn pleading patients away because the body of doctors would no longer write prescriptions for Rene's treatment for them. In December of 1939, the Commission issued its official report, which concluded:

> After a careful examination of all the evidence submitted and analyzed herewith, and not forgetting the fact that the patients, or a number of them, who came before the Commission felt that they had been benefited by the treatment which they received, the Commission is of the opinion that the evidence adduced does not justify any favourable conclusion as to the merits of "Essiac" as a remedy for cancer, and would so report. (Glum 1988, 91)

Although the Commission could draw no favorable conclusions about Essiac from their formal investigation, it is interesting to note that their interest in Essiac's formulation had not diminished. This is evidenced by the last paragraph of the Commission's report:

> If, however, Miss Caisse is desirous of having her treatment further investigated, and wishes to submit thereon further evidence, and is prepared to furnish the Commission with the formula of "Essiac" together with samples thereof (a fourth request), the Commission will be glad to make such investigation, in such manner as is deemed desirable and warranted. (Glum 1988, 91)

The report was front-page news throughout Canada. The press made much of the fact that the report stated that of the forty-nine patients who testified at the hearing, only four of the diagnoses were accepted as valid by the Commission. The other forty-five cases were dismissed on these bases: the original diagnoses of cancer had been incorrect (seemingly an indictment of their own ranks); the patients' cancer had been healed by previous radium or X-ray treatments; or doctors had written letters disavowing a patient's diagnosis. Further, the report implied that "only" forty-nine patients, from Rene's large practice came forward to testify. It made no mention of the additional three hundred thirty-eight individuals ready to testify who were waiting in the ballroom, but denied a chance to speak before the Committee. It was also implicit in the report that the patients themselves were somehow mistaken about their own cases. It is amazing how three hundred thirty-eight patients, plus forty-nine testifying patients, and their doctors could be so wrong about their cancer diagnoses.

Rene Caisse defended herself and countered the Committee's findings in writing with all the facts she could gather. She also wrote to Premier Hepburn. Her letters were all published in the newspapers, but nothing became of them. She continued to treat those who had prescriptions, but there were not many. She was devastated by the hostility of the medical establishment after all her years of collaborating with them, and she worried that she would be prosecuted under the Kirby Bill. So, in January of 1941, she made the heartbreaking decision to close her clinic.

In her farewell statement, she said one of the most important things she had ever stated during her career as a nurse:

"I am proud of my discovery of Essiac, and I believe firmly in [my] heart that someday, on its merit, Essiac will be recognized and made available to all cancer sufferers the world over" (Ivey 2004, 218). Rene was near nervous collapse and suffering from exhaustion. After this final closing of her clinic, she returned to North Bay to be with her husband Charles and his family.

Rene removed herself from public view and led a quiet life in North Bay. Charles died of pneumonia in 1943 at age fifty-seven. Rene took his death very hard and became even more reclusive. Little is known or written about her during the fifteen years that followed Charles's death. It is speculated that she continued to brew small amounts of Essiac, but because she was still being watched by the Cancer Commission, she had to treat the few cancer patients that came to her surreptitiously.

In 1958, the Cancer Commission recommended that Rene Caisse's activities be looked into by the College of Physicians and Surgeons. Apparently, the public was again becoming vocal in their support of Nurse Caisse and her treatment.

In 1959, a former patient of Rene's, Roland Davidson, who had been cured of acute ulcerated hemorrhoids many years before, decided to make it his mission to have Essiac recognized once and for all. He approached Ralph Daigh, the President of Fawcett Publications, about printing a story on Essiac and its founder, Rene Caisse. He was armed with documentation that spanned thirty years. Mr. Daigh was most impressed, but decided to arrange for further investigation of Essiac, so that this time there could be no question as to its merit. He arranged for Rene to do further research under the supervision of Dr. Charles Brusch, at the Brusch Medical Center in Cambridge, Massachusetts.

Dr. Charles Brusch was a highly respected physician with credentials and honors too numerous to list in entirety. He was the personal physician of President John F. Kennedy. He was the doctor who administered the first polio vaccination in the United States. He and his brother headed the Brusch Medical Center, the largest medical clinic in Massachusetts. He was considered a great humanitarian and visionary. He believed in preventative medicine, and he had done some research into acupuncture. He initiated a program at his clinic to help those too poor to pay for treatment. He was very interested in Essiac and its merits, and he welcomed the opportunity to work with Rene Caisse, who was now seventy years old.

Rene was thrilled with the collaboration. She would be able to test Essiac on human cancer sufferers under the guidance of a man she hugely respected. Along with Dr. Brusch, she would also be supervised by the Director of Research, Dr. Charles McClure. After only three months, Drs. Brusch and McClure would issue their first report, which stated:

> Clinically, on patients suffering from pathologically proven cancer, it reduces pain and causes a recession in the growth; patients have gained weight and shown an improvement in their general health.
>
> This after only three months' tests, and proof Miss Caisse has to show of the many patients she has benefited in the past twenty-five years, has convinced the doctors at Brusch Medical Center that Essiac has merit in the treatment of cancer. The doctors do not say that Essiac is a cure, but they do say it is a benefit. It is non-toxic, and is administered both orally and by intramuscular injection. (Thomas 1993, 37-38)

As part of the research effort, Dr. Brusch advised Rene to contact former patients and ask them to fill out a questionnaire. He wanted to determine their long-term survival rates. They sent properly witnessed, written testimonials to Rene and Dr. Brusch. Their testimonies seem to validate Rene's belief that Essiac could indeed cure cancer. The patients all reported being alive and well and having no recurrence of cancer:

Norma Thompson............treated 20 years ago
Clara Thornbury...............treated 22 years ago
D. H. Laundry....................treated 11 years ago
Nellie McVittee .................treated 23 years ago
Wilson Hammer ...............treated 31 years ago
John McNee .......................treated 30 years ago
Jack Finley.........................treated 20 years ago
Lizzie Ward........................treated 14 years ago
J. H. Stewart......................treated 16 years ago
Eliza Veitch .......................treated 18 years ago
Fred Walker.......................treated 20 years ago

(Thomas 1993, 39)

Dr. Brusch suggested to Rene that they further support their findings by running clinical trials on both mice and human subjects. This way, they could refine Essiac further to obtain optimal results. The Memorial Sloan-Kettering Institute in New York agreed to supply them with mice. Things continued to go well. Dr. Brusch asked Dr. Philip Merker at Memorial Sloan-Kettering to do autopsy surveys of the test mice. Very notably, Dr. Merker reported that there were very pronounced differences between the Essiac-treated mice and the control mice. In the Essiac-treated mice, the report cited "a tendency of the cancer cells to amalgamate and localize" (Olsen 1998, 19). This prompted further interest by Sloan-Kettering and the National Cancer Institute, both of whom wanted to do further testing with Essiac. Rene was agreeable until they requested the formula; then again, she refused flatly.

Dr. Brusch was supportive of Rene and did not pressure her. He said they would continue the research on their own. Things continued to go well and all of their testing supported the efficacy of Essiac. They were able to refine the oral preparation so that it could be the sole means of administration. It would never again be given intra-muscularly. This was most advantageous to patients who would be able to administer the tea themselves; they would not have to make numerous trips to the doctor for injections. This was especially advantageous to those whose health was frail.

But, as in the past, Rene's efforts would be thwarted. The labs that had been supplying them with mice now refused to do so. In a letter to Dr. Brusch, they stated, "We cannot send you a report along the outline requested for obvious reasons. We also regret to inform you that because of technical difficulties, we will be unable to process similar material in the future" (Thomas 1993, 40). To cement their dilemma, the American Medical Association informed all of its members that they were forbidden to refer their patients to Brusch, who was administering an unknown remedy. The number of test patients plunged.

This was more than Rene could bear. She had no more fight in her, so she decided to return to Bracebridge. She trusted Dr. Brusch completely with her formula, and he promised he would continue to treat patients with it when possible. He would also try to continue laboratory testing.

Dr. Brusch was a true believer in the efficacy of Essiac. He stated, "The results we obtained with thousands of patients of various races, sexes, and ages with all types of cancer definitely prove Essiac to be a cure for cancer" (Olson 1998, 19). He demonstrated his complete confidence in Essiac in 1984, when he himself was diagnosed with cancer. In a "To Whom It May Concern" letter, signed, witnessed, and notarized, dated April 6, 1990, Dr. Brusch writes:

Many years have gone by since I first experienced the use of ESSIAC with my patients who were suffering from many forms of Cancer.

I personally monitored the use of this old therapy along with Rene Caisse RN whose many successes were widely reported. Rene worked with me at my medical clinic in Cambridge, Massachusetts, and where, under the supervision of eighteen of my many medical doctors on staff, she proceeded with a series of treatments on terminal Cancer patients and laboratory mice and together we refined and perfected her formula.

On mice, it has been shown to cause a decided recession of mass and a definite change in cell formation. Clinically, on patients suffering from pathologically proven Cancer, it reduces pain and causes a recession in growth. Patients gained weight and showed a great improvement in their general health. Their elimination improved considerably and their appetite became whetted.

Remarkably beneficial results were obtained even on those cases at the "end of the road" where it proved to prolong life and the "quality" of life.

In some cases, if the tumor didn't disappear, it could be surgically removed after ESSIAC with less risk of metastases resulting in new outbreaks.

Hemorrhage has been rapidly brought under control in many difficult cases, open lesions of lip and breast responded to treatment, and patients with Cancer of the stomach have returned to normal activity among many other remembered cases. Also, intestinal burns from radiation were healed and damage replaced, and it was found to greatly improve whatever the condition.

All these patient cases were diagnosed by reputable physicians and surgeons.

I do know that I have witnessed in my clinic and know of many other cases where ESSIAC was the therapy used, a treatment which brings about restoration through destroying the tumor tissue and improving the mental outlook, which re-establishes physiological function.

I endorse the therapy even today for I have in fact cured my own Cancer, the original site of which was the lower bowel, through ESSIAC alone.

My last complete examination, where I was examined throughout the intestinal tract while hospitalized (August 1989) for a hernia problem, no sign of malignancy was found.

Medical documents validate this.

I have taken ESSIAC every day since my diagnosis (1984) and my recent examination has given me a clean bill of health. I remained a partner with Rene Caisse until her death in 1978, and I was the only person who had her complete trust and to whom she confided her knowledge and "know-how" of what she named "ESSIAC."

Others have imitated, but a minor success rate should never be accepted when the true therapy is available.

Executed as a legal document. (Thomas 1993, Appendix/Exhibit 4)

Rene spent her retirement years in Bracebridge enjoying family and indulging in her interests of oil painting and bead making. She spent a good deal of time with her close friend, Mary McPherson. Mary had collected signatures for petitions supporting Rene and Essiac in the early years. "Both she (Mary) and her husband were successfully treated for cancer with ESSIAC in the 1940s. Always a loyal friend, she became a regular visitor at Rene's home after her retirement in 1969" (Snow and Klein 1999, 33).

Rene lived from the proceeds of the sale of some family properties and from profits from the sale of her patented kidney remedy. "Rene was still making and selling her red kidney pills, and each year federal registration No. 20027 was renewed. Back in 1951, the remedy became known as R. M. C. Kidney Tablets. Her patients found that their backaches were eased because the herbal tablets were compounded to increase the flow of urine and relieve bladder discomfort" (Ivey 2004, 239).

She still treated patients when possible, but grew more weary and suspicious of the authorities as she aged. Cancer patients still found their way to her door, but she was forced to turn many away. Her tremendous weight also caused her numerous medical problems of her own. She suffered from severe arthritis and swollen limbs, which dictated the use of a cane or wheelchair. In the beginning of her retirement, she often wintered in St. Petersburg, Florida, but as time progressed, she became mostly housebound in Bracebridge.

For some reason in 1973, Rene, at age eighty-five, again contacted Sloan-Kettering, to see if they would like to test Essiac, in light of the promising results they had received in 1959. Why Rene initiated this contact with her past adversary is unclear. It was speculated that perhaps she feared her life was drawing to a close, and she wanted her remedy to be validated before her passing. Dr. Chester Stock agreed to the testing, which took place through 1976.

This was an ill-fated alliance. The test results were disappointing, and it was later discovered that the herbs were mishandled by the lab. The herbs were ground and then suspended in sterile water and refrigerated. This was never part of the procedure. Further, Rene admitted to divulging the identity of only one of the herbs in Essiac and sending it to Dr. Stock—the herb that she felt was responsible for tumor regression. The motivations of both parties involved were unclear.

In 1977, a very popular Canadian publication, *Homemaker's Magazine*, published an extensive story on the history of Essiac and its founder, Rene Caisse. It chronicled nearly every aspect of Rene's achievements and struggles, and was replete with testimonies and authentication of

Essiac's effectiveness. The June/July/August 1977 edition of *Homemaker's Magazine* contained the article, entitled, "Could Essiac Halt Cancer?" They opened the story with this paragraph:

> Essentially, Rene's story was true. She had been getting remarkable results against many kinds of cancer with Essiac, and she had been prevented from carrying on treatment unless she revealed the formula. Whether it would have been swept under the rug by a jealous medical hierarchy, as she feared, or hailed by a grateful profession that heaped honors at her door, is a question that no one can answer, since Essiac never stood the test of controlled clinical studies. (Thomas 1993, 42)

The editorial staff of the magazine was so inspired by Rene's struggle that they came up with the idea of establishing a trust to help Rene deal with the bureaucracy and get a patent for Essiac. Rene conferred with Dr. Brusch, who urged her to accept the offer. They drew up a proposal, which Rene considered for several days, but ultimately rejected. Her objection was to the fact that six people would have to be privy to the formula. Their frustration and disappointment is evident in the closing paragraphs of their Essiac article:

> There's a tragic and shameful irony in the Essiac tale. In the beginning, a simple herbal recipe was freely shared by an Indian who understood that the blessings of the Creator belong to all.
> In the hands of more sophisticated (and allegedly more 'civilized') healers, it was made the focus of an ugly

struggle for ownership and power. Perhaps our cure for cancer lies back in the past, with our discarded humility and innocence. Perhaps the Indians will someday revive an old man's wisdom, and share it once again. Perhaps this story will be a catalyst; if so, our efforts will not have been in vain. (Thomas 1993, 42)

In August of 1977, Rene, determined not to let the secret of Essiac die with her, contacted "a lady of impeccable distinction, Ontario's Lieutenant-Governor Pauline M. McGibbon, to accept the secret formula in a sealed envelope and hold it until after Rene's death" (Ivey 2004, 262). The lieutenant governor personally came to collect the envelope and promptly had it placed in her personal safety deposit box at the Royal Bank.

The *Homemaker's Magazine* article generated an unbelievable amount of attention for Rene. Her phone never stopped ringing, and she was even the subject of a television documentary. The Essiac story was of particular interest to David Finguard of the Resperin Corporation of Toronto, a company with pharmaceutical interests. He was determined to bring Essiac to market. He visited Rene daily, sweetening his offer with every visit. He promised testing on humans and huge financial backing to bring the treatment to "suffering humanity." As always, she refused, until one day he promised that if exclusive rights for Essiac were transferred to Resperin Corporation, he would promise to open five clinics across Canada to treat terminally ill cancer patients. Those who were poor would be treated free of charge. Rene, now age eighty-nine, consulted Dr. Brusch. He agreed that it was the best offer she had received. Rene signed over the formula for Essiac to Resperin Corporation on October 26, 1977. The contract was witnessed by Dr. Brusch.

The Essiac formula given to Resperin by Rene Caisse was next officially registered by the Department of Health and Welfare as an experimental drug available for the treatment of patients with terminal cancer. It also received approval from the Health Protection Branch of the Department.

There seemed to be a general elation from the public. The management of Resperin felt a bright future was ahead. David Finguard stated, "Essiac is one of the greatest discoveries in modern science. We have found certified cases of cancer ranging over a period of twenty to thirty years, which have been cured by Essiac" (Thomas 1993, 45).

But, as if cursed, all would not go as planned once again. Two of the hospitals that were to collaborate with Resperin planned to change the protocol. They would no longer administer Essiac as the sole therapy. They wanted to use it in conjunction with other therapies that their doctors deemed necessary. There would be no way to determine Essiac's effects. Next, the Health Protection Branch of the Department of Health and Welfare decided that Resperin could no longer use the two hospitals for testing, and that testing would have to be done by private physicians. Finally, the private physicians, initially enthusiastic about the trials, found it difficult to adhere to the strict guidelines imposed by the department.

To make matters worse, the Canadian Medical Association Journal published a negative statement about Essiac. Two doctors reported that any improvements that they had seen in their patients treated with Essiac were purely subjective and possibly the results of the placebo effect. "It was presented in the CMA *Journal* as a sidebar regarding Essiac in an explosive feature report about Laetrile by Charlotte Gray, and was pointed out as another 'quack cancer cure'" (Ivey 2004, 269).

Rene spent her final year of life watching Resperin take over her struggle. On October 14, 1978, she slipped and fell, fracturing her hip. She was hospitalized in Toronto, but was never able to recover from her injury. She requested that she be moved to her hometown hospital. She died quietly in the Bracebridge hospital on December 26, 1978, at age ninety.

As time passed, it became evident that Resperin was not the pharmaceutical giant it had led Rene and Dr. Brusch to believe. They folded like a house of cards under the critical pressure applied to them in the following years. Dr. Brusch felt disillusioned with Resperin, although he did acknowledge that they were operating in a hostile environment. The Health Protection Branch accused Resperin of conducting poor clinical studies and producing results that could not be interpreted accurately.

On April 9, 1981, the Health Protection Branch explained its intentions via a lengthy internal memo to its members, which enumerated the inadequacies of Resperin's clinical research. In conclusion, the memorandum states:

> In view of this, the Health Protection Branch, on behalf of the Minister, pursuant to Section C. 08. 005 (3) intends to notify the Resperin Corporation that in the interest of public health, the clearance of the investigational new drug submission for Essiac will be cancelled.
>
> It can be expected that this decision will give rise to some accusations that the medical establishment is

not prepared to give the drug manufacturer a proper opportunity to establish its therapeutic value. There may also be a negative reaction from cancer victims who are presently taking Essiac and will have their supply cut off. Conversely, the decision will still criticism from the medical profession that the Branch is allowing an unproven drug to be distributed under inappropriate conditions. (Thomas 1993, Appendix/Exhibit 7)

There was, as predicted, huge public outrage from patients and some doctors. To quell the firestorm, the Department of Health and Welfare enacted the Emergency Drug Release Act. Under this act, a terminal patient would be allowed an unapproved medication for compassionate reasons, if his doctor provided official recommendation. However, Essiac would never again be marketed as a drug in North America.

Books have been written on Essiac, and its history has been delved into deeply. It has been the subject of radio talk shows and newspaper articles. Many facts have been compiled from the documents that Rene collected during her lifetime. Some people have claimed to be in possession of Rene's handwritten formula. Others, including Rene's trusted friend, Mary McPherson, Dr. Brusch, and the Resperin Corporation really did have the formula. Soon after Essiac's status as a drug was revoked, the formula became a matter of public record.

In December 1994, Bracebridge had a formal ceremony publicly recording the Essiac formula. A sworn affidavit signed by Mary McPherson and the hand-written formula with its instructions for brewing are still displayed today in a Bracebridge Museum room dedicated to Rene Caisse. To further honor Rene, Bracebridge named a street after her (Rene Caisse Lane) and erected a bronze statue of her.

Because it was clear that the demand for Essiac would never go away, and that it could no longer be classified as a drug, a new avenue for distribution of the herbal remedy evolved. It is now marketed as a non-toxic herbal tea, and is widely available throughout Canada, the United States, and many parts of the world. It is a natural food product, so is easily distributed by health food stores and the like. It can be purchased in person, by mail, and over the Internet. It is sold under many names, by many different manufacturers, most claiming to use Rene's original formulation. The herbs can be purchased in dry form, for customers to brew themselves, or as a pre-brewed tea in glass bottles. No manufacturer can make any medical claims regarding this product, although most customers are already aware of Essiac's history when they purchase it.

# THE ESSIAC HERBS AND RECIPE

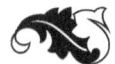

By some accounts, the Indian recipe given to Rene by the elderly Englishwoman contained eight herbs. Supposedly, during the years that Rene refined her recipe, she deleted four of the herbs. Only three of the four omitted herbs are named in any documentation. They are periwinkle, watercress, and red clover. However, the Essiac tea recipe used by Rene Caisse, as authenticated by her friend, Mary McPherson, and other Essiac researchers, contains the following four herbs: burdock root, sheep sorrel, slippery elm bark, and turkey rhubarb root. These four herbs are the ones used in most formulations available today, but some manufacturers add additional herbs, which they claim enhance the original formula. A description of each of the original four herbs follows.

**Burdock Root:** Its Latin name is *Arctium lappa*, and it is a member of the *Asteraceae* family. Other relatives include thistle, sunflower, echinacea, and dandelion. Burdock is a biennial, considered a weed, and is prolific throughout the United States and Canada. It was brought to North America by early settlers from Europe and Asia. It has been used medicinally in China for over two thousand years. "Hildegard of Bingen, a twelfth century German abbess, considered burdock a valuable remedy for cancerous tumors. Herbalists in other cultures and times, including the Americas, China, India, and Russia have turned to the root of this familiar herb for the folk treatment of cancer" (Hanrahan 2001). It is used as a food product called gobo in Japan and Hawaii. All parts of the plant are edible and used for various reasons, but the root is considered to have medicinal value. Only the root of the burdock plant is used in Essiac tea.

In her authoritative guide to herbs and herbal preparations, Phyllis A. Balch, CNC, cites the following benefits of burdock root use:

> As a blood purifier, burdock clears congestion in circulatory, lymphatic, respiratory, and urinary systems. It can help eliminate excess fluids in the body and stimulate the elimination of toxic waste materials, which relieves liver disorders and improves digestion. It cleanses the body of bile and detoxifies the kidneys and gallbladder. It increases perspiration, which also reduces excess toxins. Herbalists recognize its ability to prevent surging and sinking blood-sugar levels, detoxify the liver, and act against cancer.

In traditional Chinese medicine (TCM), burdock root is used in combination with other herbs to treat sore throats, tonsillitis, colds, and measles. (Balch 2002, 38)

Most herbal references ascribe the above attributes to burdock root, and some mention burdock as being mildly warming and moisturizing. In China, it is also considered a rejuvenating tonic and an aphrodisiac. *Arctium Lappa*'s uses are listed by Tierra (2003): "[It is used] for various types of cancers including breast, lungs, and gastrointestinal. It is detoxifying, diuretic, nutritive, and desmutagenic (prevents cellular mutation)" (Tierra 2003, 87).

**Sheep Sorrel**: Its Latin name is *Rumex acetosella*, and it's a member of the *polygonaceae* or buckwheat family. It is a perennial plant that flourishes in England, but it grows worldwide, except for the tropics. Native Americans used all parts of the plant as food and as medicine. It has been used to stop hemorrhages because of its astringent properties, as well as its vitamin K content. (Vitamin K helps the blood to clot properly.) The entire plant is ground for use in Essiac tea.

Herbal references refer to sheep sorrel's use in the treatment of many types of cancer. One text lists the following therapeutic actions:

The whole herb, when young and in its freshest state, acts as a diuretic and [as a] blood cleanser. The herb improves liver, intestinal, and bowel functions; prevents the destruction of red blood cells; and is used to break down tumors. The chlorophyll in sheep sorrel leaves carries oxygen through the bloodstream, which strengthens cell walls, helps remove deposits in blood vessels and allows the body to store and use more oxygen. Chlorophyll may also reduce radiation damage and restrict chromosome damage. The herb is smooth and acid while the root has astringent properties and contains a substance allied to crysophanic acid (an iron-greening tannin diuretic). Sheep sorrel is taken for inflammatory diseases, tumors, incipient cancers, and urine and kidney diseases. The action is refrigerant, diaphoretic, and diuretic. (Olson 1998, 49)

Rene Caisse always maintained that only one of the herbs in her Essiac formula was responsible for tumor regression, with the others playing supportive roles as detoxifiers and immune strengtheners. That one herb she referred to is sheep sorrel.

Of the four herbs in the recipe, the quality of the sheep sorrel seems to be the deciding factor as to the overall effectiveness of the Essiac formula, and it was the one herb that Rene isolated during her early years of research as having a direct effect on cancerous tumors. (Snow and Klein 1999, 22)

Of the four Essiac herbs, sheep sorrel is the least easily harvested in large commercial quantities while maintaining quality. Unscrupulous or irresponsible herb suppliers may try to substitute other easily harvested dock plants, such as yellow dock (*rumex crispus*) or broad-leaved dock (*rumex obtusifolius*). A consumer must find a trusted company that can guarantee they use only true sheep sorrel (*rumex acetosella*).

**Slippery Elm Bark**: Its Latin name is *Ulmus rubra*, formerly *Ulmus fulva*. It's a member of the elm family, and is sometimes called red elm, moose elm, sweet elm, or Indian elm. It is a large deciduous tree native to the North American continent. The inner bark of the trunk and branches is used medicinally. This bark was used extensively by the Native Americans: topically for wounds, as a gruel to feed the sick, and as a preservative for meat.

Balch (2002) cites evidence of the benefits of slippery elm bark for the following ailments:

> Slippery elm has a soothing and healing effect on any part of the body it comes into contact with. It is used in the treatment of sore throats, indigestion, digestive irritation, and stomach ulcers. It is able to neutralize excess acids in the stomach and intestines. It can also be used externally to heal wounds and burns, and can relieve irritated, inflamed, or itchy skin. The mucilage in slippery elm bark is an excellent remedy for irritation and inflammation of the reproductive and respiratory systems, as well as the urinary tract. (Balch 2002, 127)

The slippery elm tree, along with its other family members, was nearly wiped out by Dutch elm disease. This devastating disease was carried by the elm bark beetle in a log imported from England during the 1930s. Fortunately, the elms are making a comeback. Only the bark of the slippery elm is used in the making of Essiac tea. Reputable suppliers harvest the bark in a manner that does not harm the tree.

**Turkey Rhubarb**: Its Latin name is *Rheum palmatum* of the *polygonaceae* family. It is an ornamental perennial, sometimes called Chinese rhubarb. It originated in western China and Tibet and spread throughout Europe. It was imported to North America by European settlers. Today it is imported from Russia and China and cultivated in many places around the world. Documentation shows that it was used by Chinese and Greek physicians. Unlike the milder domestic rhubarb (*rheum rhaponticum*), turkey rhubarb root has strong medicinal value. Only the powdered root is used in the making of Essiac.

Several herbal reference guides cite Turkey rhubarb as a cancer remedy. Michael Tierra specifically mentions its use "for colorectal cancer, uterine and ovarian cancer, and granulocytic leukemia" (Tierra 2003, 93). Olson (1998) describes its therapeutic action as follows:

> Turkey rhubarb has been used for centuries for its dual action as a laxative and astringent as well as a purging treatment. In smaller doses, it's used to treat diarrhea or to stimulate the appetite. Larger amounts yield a laxative effect. The herb stimulates the colon and abates distension while promoting bile flow, clearing stasis, and restoring the stomach and liver. It has been used as a stomach tonic to soothe digestion; to cleanse the liver; as an anti-tumor; and an aid for thermal burns, jaundice, sores, and cancers. (51-52)

Essiac is a decoction, which simply means a preparation made by boiling a substance to extract properties from its original form. Publications by Ivey (2004), Olsen (1998), Percival (1994), and Snow and Klein (2001), all contain Rene Caisse's recipe for the Essiac decoction, as confirmed and authenticated by Mary McPherson. In addition to listing the four component herbs, they also list the measurements.

Confusion arises because sometimes the amount of burdock used is referred to by volume instead of weight, whereas the measurement for the other three ingredients is always listed by weight. Below the authentic Essiac recipe is given using Imperial and Metric measure, as well as volume for burdock root:

### US/Canada/Imperial/Metric
6.5 US cups (24oz/680g) Burdock root, chopped to the size of small peas
16 ounces (453g) powdered Sheep sorrel
4 ounces (113g) powdered Slippery elm bark
1 ounces (28.35g) powdered Turkey rhubarb root
(Snow and Klein 2001, 14)

Mary McPherson knew Rene Caisse for a period of forty-three years. They had a strong friendship, and Mary often helped Rene brew her tea in Rene's later years. The sworn affidavit that Mary McPherson gave to the town of Bracebridge for public record in 1994 included the recipe for Essiac and Mary's handwritten instructions for preparation of the tea, entitled "Exhibit A." These documents are kept safe in the Bracebridge Library, the town's archives, and the Bracebridge Historical Society. Her instructions follow:

Take a measuring cup, use 1 ounce of herb mixture to 32 ounces of water depending on the amount you want to make.

I use 1 cup of mixture to 8 x 32 = 256 ounces of water. Boil hard for ten minutes (covered), then turn off but leave sitting on warm plate overnight (cooling).

In the morning, heat to steaming hot and let sit a few minutes. Then strain through fine strainer into hot sterilized bottles and sit to cool in dark cool cupboard.

When it's thick, pour into a large jar, and let it sit in fridge overnight, and then pour off all you can without sediment.

It must be refrigerated when opened.

The recipe must be followed exactly as written. I use a granite preserving kettle 10-12 quarts, an 8-ounce measuring cup, a small funnel, and a fine strainer to fill the bottles. (Ivey 2004, 304-305)

Rene diluted one ounce of Essiac with an ounce of hot water and had her patients drink it as a tea. Today, Essiac users typically take a dosage of one to six ounces daily depending on their conditions and reasons for using Essiac. For example, someone wanting to take Essiac as a tonic for general health or prophylactically for cancer prevention might take one ounce daily. Whereas, an individual with advanced cancer may take three two-ounce doses divided throughout the day. It is best taken on an empty stomach.

It is cautioned that Essiac herbs never be frozen, and the tea never microwaved. If mold ever forms in the bottles or on the dry herbs, those should be discarded immediately. This situation can arise due to improper storage or lack of sterilization. Users can purchase dry herbs and make their own decoction or buy it pre-brewed in sterilized glass bottles.

# INVESTIGATION AND EFFICACY OF ESSIAC

T hus far, the volume of evidence of Essiac's benefit in the treatment of cancer patients is impressive to say the least: doctor-signed petitions, petitions signed by citizens (one with fifty-five thousand signatures), public endorsements by prestigious doctors (Dr. Frederick Banting, Dr. Emma M. Carson, and Dr. Charles Brusch), and hundreds of personal testimonies. The fact that a woman would devote fifty years of her life to treating terminal cancer patients without financial gain is probably the ultimate testimony to Essiac.

Rene Caisse and Essiac have been the subject of newspaper and magazine articles, a television documentary, radio talk shows, and a half dozen books. Essiac has been used by cancer patients for over ninety years. It is estimated that up to twenty thousand North American cancer patients may be currently taking an Essiac-like tea. (Boik 2003)

However impressive this all seems, it is still considered anecdotal evidence. With the exception of Rene's early mice experiments, Memorial Sloan-Kettering's review of mice autopsy surveys, and reports written at the Brusch Medical Center, little clinical proof was published during Rene's lifetime. Rene would argue that all of her patients were clinical proof, but Western medicine during the last century is loath to acknowledge any unproven therapy, no matter the volume of anecdotal evidence. A therapy is considered unproven if it has not met the rigors of hard science. A valid therapy must be evaluated clinically and documented with published results.

With one exception, the clinical research on Essiac, or any of its component herbs, has been minimal. The following is a chronology of investigations into Essiac and its component herbs:

**In 1952,** researchers Belkin and Fitzgerald published a study in *The Journal of the National Cancer Institute* regarding the tumor-damaging capacity of plant materials. In it, they noted that *Rheum palmatum* (turkey rhubarb) "has been demonstrated to have antitumor activity in the sarcoma thirty-seven test system" (Snow and Klein 1999, 31).

**In 1966,** *Tumori*, a journal of experimental and clinical oncology, published the findings of two Hungarian scientists from the University of Szeged. They reported findings of antitumor activity in a purified fraction of Arctium lappa (burdock). Burdock was included in their study because of its prevalence of use as a folk remedy (Dombradi and Foldeak 1966).

**In 1978,** The Resperin Corporation filed a preclinical new drug submission with the Canadian Department of

Health and Welfare. At that time, they were given permission to conduct safety and efficacy studies on Essiac in cancer patients. In 1982, the Department rescinded its permission, claiming that the research was not being conducted as originally planned. (Recall from the history portion of this work that the Department of Health would not allow two hospitals to participate in the studies, and they put stringent restrictions on doctors participating in the study. Further, Essiac was never allowed to be the sole form of treatment, making it impossible to determine its contribution to outcome.) This may explain why the research was not being conducted as originally planned. It was concluded that:

> At that time [1982], the available incomplete data were reviewed, and no clear evidence of improved survival could be demonstrated for treated patients. Pain control and quality of life were not assessed in these studies. The review of the data indicated, however, that Essiac was not toxic. (National Cancer Institute 2005, para. 2)

In 1984, researchers from the Nagoya University in Japan isolated a desmutagan in burdock. A desmutagen is a substance that is capable of reducing the extent or frequency of a genetic mutation. Genetic mutation can initiate cancers. They named this isolated substance the B-factor. Their findings are as follows:

> A desmutagenic factor was isolated from burdock (Arctum lappa Linne). This factor reduced the mutagenicity of mutagens that are active without metabolic activation, such as 4-NO2-1, 2-DAB and 2-NO2-1, and

4-DAB, as well as mutagens such as ethidium bromide, 2-aminoanthracene, Trp-P-1 and Trp-P-2 requiring S9 for metabolic activation. It is resistant to heat and proteolytic enzymes and sensitive to treatment with MnC12. The partially purified principles had molecular weight higher than 300,000 [sic] and showed characteristics of a polyanionic substance. An irreversible diminution of the mutagen was confirmed by treatment of 2-NO2-1, 4-DAB, or Trp-P-2 with the burdock factor. (Morita et al. 1984, 25)

**In 1996,** Chinese researchers, at Kaohsiung Medical College in Taiwan investigated Arctium lappa for anti-inflammatory and free radical scavenger activity. Inflammation and free radical overload are implicated in cell mutation and cancer development. Their findings are as follows:

The effects of Arctium lappa L. (root) on anti-inflammatory and free radical activity were investigated. Subcutaneous administration of A. lappa crude extract significantly decreased carrageenan-induced rat paw edema. When simultaneously treated with CC14, it produced pronounced activities against CC14-induced acute liver damage. The free radical scavenging activity of its crude extract was also examined by means of an electron spin resonance (ERS) spectrometer. The IC50 of A. lappa extract on superoxide and hydroxyl radical scavenger activity was 2.06 mg/ml and 11.8 mg/ml, respectively. These findings suggest that Arctium lappa possess free radical scavenging activity. The inhibitory effects on carrageenan-induced paw edema and

CC14-induced hepatotoxicity could be due to the scavenging effect of A. lappa. (Lin et al. 1996, 127)

In 1998, Elizabeth Kaegi, MB, ChB, MSc, wrote a series of articles on unconventional therapies for cancer. She did this on behalf of the Task Force on Alternative Therapies of the Canadian Breast Cancer Research Initiative. The first therapy that she evaluated was Essiac. Her article was lengthy, mostly summarizing Essiac's history. As far as use and safety of Essiac, she states,

> Proponents advise that Essiac is compatible with all other cancer treatments, including chemotherapy and radiotherapy. Most people trying Essiac today use it in addition to conventional treatments or as a component of care for terminal disease. Adverse effects associated with the use of Essiac have not been reported. (Kaegi 1998, 900)

She found no randomized controlled clinical trials or case-controlled studies on Essiac, but reported the following on the constituent herbs:

> A number of laboratory studies of burdock root and Indian rhubarb were found. Both of these herbs have a long history of use as folk medicines and are included in many compendia of herbal remedies, being valued for their properties as laxatives, promoters of wound healing, and folk remedies for cancer. They contain relatively high concentrations of flavones, anthraquinones, tannins, and certain polysaccharides, which have been variously reported to have antioxidant, immunomodulatory, antimutagenic and cytostatic effects.

Interestingly, a number of conventional chemothera-
peutic agents (e.g., adriamycin) are anthraquinone
derivatives. Burdock extract caused necrosis in solid
tumours in mice and has been found to inhibit the
effects of known mutagens. (Kaegi 1998, 901)

**In 2000**, a review of the chemistry and biological activity
of the herbs used in Essiac and Flor-Essence herbal tonic was
published in the monthly journal, *Phytotherapy Research*.
Flor-Essence is a product that contains the original four
Essiac herbs; burdock root, slippery elm bark, sheep sorrel,
and turkey rhubarb, as well as red clover, blessed thistle, kelp
and watercress. The review states:

> The herbal mixtures, Essiac and Flor-Essence, are
> sold as nutritional supplements and used by patients
> to treat chronic conditions, particularly cancer.
> Evidence of anticancer activity for the herbal teas is
> limited to anecdotal reports recorded for some forty
> years in Canada. Individual case reports suggest that
> the tea improves quality of life, alleviates pain, and in
> some cases, impacts cancer progression among cancer
> patients. Experimental studies with individual herbs
> have shown evidence of biological activity including
> antioxidant, antioestrogenic, immunostimulant, anti-
> tumour, and antiocholeretic actions. However, research
> that demonstrates these positive effects in the experi-
> mental setting has not been translated to the clinical
> arena. (Tamayo et al. 2000, 1)

**In 2004**, researchers at the Center for Complementary
Medicine Research in Vancouver, British Columbia

conducted in vitro comparisons of Essiac and Flor-Essence using human tumor cell lines. Their findings were published in *Oncology Reports*. They studied these two products because of their prevalence of use by North American cancer patients during chemo and radiation therapies. They concluded, "Our data show that both ES [Essiac] and FE [Flor-Essence] herbal teas demonstrated antiproliferative and differentiation inducing properties in vitro [outside a living organism, i.e. test tube] only at high concentrations. Further research is needed to elucidate the in vivo [inside a living organism] activities" (Tai et al. 2004, 471). The study also noted that ES has higher differentiation inducing activity that FE. Differentiation and proliferation are means of measuring cancer cells formation and reproduction.

**In 2004,** researchers at Indiana University/Purdue University assessed the ability of Essiac to inhibit prostate cancer-cell proliferation. They published their findings in *The Journal of Alternative and Complementary Medicine*. A synopsis follows:

OBJECTIVE: To assess the ability of Essiac tea extracts (Essiac Canada International, Ottawa, Canada) to modulate cancer cell proliferation and immune responsiveness.

DESIGN: A noncancerous transformed cell line was compared to a cancerous cell line and spleen cells that had been isolated from mice to examine proliferation responses mediated by the addition of an Essiac preparation.

RESULTS: We found in vitro evidence of decreased proliferation of both noncancerous transformed (CHO) and cancerous prostate cell line (LNCaP) when Essiac was present in the culture media. A dose response for inhibition was demonstrated by a linear regression performed on the data for both the CHO and LNCaP cells. The percent inhibition of the LNCaP cells was higher than the percent inhibition of the CHO cells suggesting that Essiac may have a more selective effect on cancer cells than transformed cells. In addition, the effects of Essiac were examined in an immune T-lymphocyte proliferation assay. At low doses of Essiac, augmentation of proliferation of these T cells was demonstrated, but at higher doses, Essiac was inhibitory to T-cell proliferation. The same doses of Essiac that stimulated spleen cells were inhibitory for LNCaP cell proliferation.

CONCLUSIONS: Essiac preparations may be able to inhibit tumor cell growth while enhancing immune response to antigenic stimulation. This may be especially valuable in immune-suppressed individuals. (Ottenweller et al. 2004, 687)

**In 2006**, a study of Essiac was performed at the Pathology and Physiology Research Branch Health Effects Laboratory Division of the National Institute for Occupational Safety and Health. The objective of the study was to observe Essiac's effect on DNA damage and scavenging of reactive oxygen species. Reactive oxygen species, sometimes called free radicals, can damage cell membranes due to oxidative stress. Their findings are as follows:

Essiac, a tea reportedly developed by the Ojibwa tribe of Canada and widely publicized as a homeopathic cancer treatment, is prepared from a mixture of four herbs: Arctium lappa, Rumex acetosella, Ulmus rubra, and Rheum officinale. Each of these herbs has been reported to possess antioxidant and anti-cancer activity. Essiac itself has also been reported to demonstrate anti-cancer activity in vitro, although its effects in vivo are still a matter of debate. We prepared an extract of Essiac tea from a concentration of 25mg/mL and boiled it for ten minutes. From this preparation, we used concentrations of 5, 10, 25, and 50 percent to measure Essiac effects. In this study, we examined the effects of Essiac on free radical scavenging and DNA damage in a non-cellular system, as well as the effects of Essiac on lipid peroxidation using the RAW 264.7 cell line. We observed, using electron spin resonance that Essiac effectively scavenged hydroxyl, up to 84 percent reduction in radical signal at the 50 percent tea preparation concentration, and superoxide radicals, up to 82 percent reduction in radical signal at the 50 percent tea preparation concentration, as well as prevented hydroxyl radical-induced DNA damage. In addition, Essiac inhibited hydroxyl radical-induced lipid peroxidation by up to 50 percent at the 50 percent tea preparation concentration. These data indicate that Essiac tea possesses potent antioxidant and DNA-protective activity, properties that are common to natural anti-cancer agents. This study may help to explain the mechanisms behind the reported anti-cancer effects of Essiac. (Leonard et al. 2006, 288)

These ten investigations of Essiac, Essiac-like products, and its component herbs are of interest individually, but they become even more noteworthy when the results are viewed cumulatively. Patterns and commonalities emerge that beg for further examination. It was stated earlier that clinical research on Essiac has been minimal to date, with one exception.

References to Essiac research conducted in Europe and Asia (particularly China and Japan) can be found, but the studies themselves are not readily available. Most are published in foreign language journals or located in inaccessible, specialty libraries. The one exception referred to above is an elegant study conducted in China. Although the complete sixty-five-page report has yet to be translated into English, a translated summary of the clinical study that was submitted to the Chinese Ministry of Health is available. (Lui and Chan 1995a, 1995b, 1995c; Yan et al. 1996)

In the United States and Canada, the two health regulatory bodies (FDA and Health Canada, respectively), regulate herbs differently than they do medicines. This is why Essiac is marketed in North America as an herbal tonic and not a drug. In China, however, herbs are considered powerful medicines and are regulated as such by the Chinese Ministry of Health. In China, it is the norm, not the exception, for patients to be administered herbal medicine, either alone or in conjunction with other conventional treatments.

In the early 1990s, Chinese cancer sufferers became aware of Native American Indian remedies and specifically the herbs contained in the Essiac formulation. Some of the ingredients in Essiac and Essiac products were unfamiliar to China, which has long been considered the herbal kingdom of the world. The Chinese Ministry of Health required that any Essiac product would have to go through the same investigational rigors as any medicine used in China, herbal or otherwise. They agreed to conduct studies on two products manufactured in Canada and distributed by MPS International Marketing Inc. The two products are CESSIAC® and YUCCALIVE®, both registered trademarks. CESSIAC® contains the original four herbs of Essiac: burdock root, sheep sorrel, slippery elm bark, and turkey rhubarb. YUCCALIVE® contains yucca schidigera, fennel seed, anise seed, honey, licorice root, clove bud, and cinnamon bark, which are said to enhance the effectiveness of the CESSIAC® formulation.

The studies were conducted over the course of three years at three major Chinese hospitals: the Beijing Chinese Medicine University East Gate Hospital, the People's Hospital of Guangdong Province, and the Guangzhou City Cancer Hospital, in addition to the Research Section of Pharmacology, Institute of Materia Medica of Guangdong Province. The investigations conducted included toxicity test, medicinal test, tumor inhibition test, immunological test, and a clinical study of two hundred forty-five cases. (Lui and Chan 1995a, 1995b, 1995c; Yan et al. 1996)

The effectiveness of CESSIAC® and YUCCALIVE® was confirmed by the results of these studies. Based on this evidence, the Chinese Ministry of Health issued import permits in 1996 for these two medicinal herbal formulations. Most importantly, these were the first ever non-traditional Chinese medicines to be issued import permits for a Class A disease (denotes life threatening). In China, the CESSIAC® product has the registered name of Kang Ji, which means "foundation of health." YUCCALIVE® is registered as Yu Kang, which means "health's nourishment." Some specifics of the studies follow:

CESSIAC® and YUCCALIVE® are referred to as "C" Formula and "Y" Formula in the studies. A study on the tumor-inhibition effect of the combined use of formulas "C" and "Y" imported from Canada was conducted in 1993, according to the *Guidelines of Pre-clinical Study of New Chinese Medicine*, Ministry of Health of China (Lui and Chan, 1995c). The study used NIH (National Institutes of Health) mice, which had been vaccinated with mice hepatic carcinoma (cancer strain) subcutaneously (under the skin).

The mice were divided into five groups according to weight. Three groups were gastro-fed with the "C" formula first, and then the "Y" one hour later. The first group received a low dose, the second an intermediate dose, and the third a high dose. The other two groups of mice were contrast groups; one was fed physiological saline, the other 5-FU (a chemotherapy agent), and no "C" or "Y" formulas. The mice were treated this way for ten consecutive days, and on the eleventh day, they were killed. Tumor masses were removed and weighed. A statistical analysis was performed to determine the tumor inhibition rate (TIR). As per the clinical guidelines, the test was conducted three times.

According to the Research Section of Pharmacology, Institute of Materia Medica of Guangdong Province, the results were as follows:

> For the group of intermediate dosage, the tumor-inhibi-
> tion rate was greater than 30 percent for all three tests.
> In addition, for every test, the results were significant
> or notably significant compared to those of the physi-
> ological saline group. For the high dosage group, only
> the first test had a tumor-inhibition rate lower than 30

percent, but the results were significant for all three tests. For the low dosage group, the tumor-inhibition rate of the first test was lower than 30 percent and was not statistically significant. However, for the other two tests, the tumor-inhibition rate was greater than 30 percent, and also significant statistically. (Lui and Chan 1995c, Results)

Further, the following two discussions are presented in the research results:

According to *Guidelines on Pre-clinical Study of New Chinese Medicine*, if a drug has a statistically significant tumor-inhibition rate of 30 percent on an animal transplantation tumor, the drug is classified as having tumor-inhibition effect. The current laboratory study has shown that the combined use of "C" Formula and "Y" Formula had notable tumor-inhibition effects, with the intermediate dosage group being the most significant [Test 1: 30 percent, Test 2: 35.5 percent and Test 3: 47 percent]. The tumor-inhibition rate of high dosage group was slightly lower than that of the intermediate group, but the difference was not statistically significant. This indicates that increasing dosage does not increase the tumor inhibition effect.

During the laboratory test, the cancer-carrying mice undergoing treatment of the two drugs had better general appearance, activity level, and appetite compared to the negative contrast group, indicating that the combined use of the two drugs can also improve the general status of the cancer-carrying animals, i.e., improve the quality of their lives. (Lui and Chan 1995c, Results)

Acute Toxicity Tests were also conducted on "C" Formula and "Y" Formula at the Guangdong Provincial Institute of Materia Medica with the objective of observing the acute toxic reaction of white mice following the oral administration of "C" Formula and "Y" Formula. The procedure and result of "C" Formula testing is as follows:

1.  <u>Treatment of medicine</u>: Condense 1,000 ml of "C" Formula into 20 ml over double boiler to be used in experiment.
2.  <u>Acute Toxicity Test</u>: Select thirty white mice between 20 to 22 g each, fifteen male and fifteen female. Mouth feed mice with condensed Formula according to 0.4ml/10g (equivalent to the strength of 2,000 ml/kg of the original medicine) all at once. Observed continuously for seven days after feeding. All mice survived with normal appetite and vitality. It is concluded that the mice can take up to 2,000 ml/kg of "C" Formula. This dosage is equivalent to 555 times of the normal daily dosage of an adult or 1,666 times of one normal dosage of an adult.

It is concluded that oral administration of the "C" Formula is safe. (Lui and Chan 1995a, Experimental Procedure and Results)

The procedure and result of Y Formula testing is as follows:

1.  Medicine Treatment: Condense 1,000 ml of "Y" Formula into 100 ml over double boiler to be used in experiment.

2. Acute Toxicity test through oral administration on mouse: select thirty mice weight between 20 to 22 g fifteen MALE and fifteen FEMALE. Feed mice with the entire dosage condensed Formula (equivalent to the strength of 70.61 ml/kg of the original medicine). Observe mice for seven days after feeding. All mice survived with a normal appetite. It is observed that the mice can take up to 70.61 ml/kg of "Y" Formula orally without any problem. (For an average adult of 50 kg in China, normal dosage is 30 ml per day orally.) The dosage is this test is equivalent to 117 times of the normal dosage. The dosage of 20 ml per day per adult is recommended for clinical testing.

It is concluded that oral administration of the "Y" Formula is safe. (Lui and Chan, 1995b, Experimental Procedure and Results)

In addition to the study on tumor-inhibition and the acute toxicity testing, a Clinical Report on the Therapeutic Effect of "C" Formula and "Y" Formula from thirty-nine cases was prepared (Yan et al. 1996). The thirty-nine cases were selected from Guangdong Province based on guidelines of clinical research, which are specified in the Law of Medicine Anticancer Drugs. Of the thirty-nine subjects, twenty-three were cancer patients, and sixteen were patients having idiopathic and secondary immunological deficiency diseases caused by an imbalance of the immunologic system.

All of the cancer patients had diagnoses confirmed by pathological histology, cytologic diagnosis, or definite marks of tumors. Their types of cancer were diverse: nasopharyneal carcinoma, hepatic carcinoma, carcinoma of the colon, metracarcinoma, mammary cancer, adrenal tumor hepar metastasis, carcinoma ventri culi, hepatic cyst, and gall polypus. The average age of the patients was 48.6, and ten of the cancer patients were female and thirteen male.

The immune deficiency patients included the following: chronic persistent hepatitis, rhinallergosis, pulmonary tuberculosis, coronary heart disease, and diabetes. Of these cases, five were male and eleven female, with an average age of forty.

With the exception of three cancer patients who were in advanced stage of multiple and metastatic type, all related drugs were discontinued to effectively test "C" Formula and "Y" Formula. The tumor patients were administered the two test drugs orally at the following dosage:

> "C" Formula: 90 ml T.I.D. (three times per day) x 90 days
> "Y" Formula: 20 ml B.I.D. (two times per day) x 90 days

The Immunologic deficiency patients were administered the two test drugs orally at the following dosage:

> "C" Formula: 60 ml B.I.D. x 30 days or
> 90 ml B.I.D. x 30 days
> "Y" Formula: 30 ml Q.D. (every day) x 30 days

The discussion from the report's conclusion follows:

Of the thirty-nine cases in this group of study, twenty-three were tumor patients, and sixteen were secondary immunologic deficiency patients. Among the twenty-three tumor patients, three died of advanced metastatic carcinoma since they had been already at critical stage when starting the current treatment. There was one case of complete remission, six cases of partial remission, and thirteen cases of moderate remission and stabilized development. The total remission rate was 30.43 percent. The rate of moderate remission and stabilized development was 56.52 percent. The death rate was 13.04 percent.

Of the sixteen secondary immunologic deficiency cases, five were notably effective, eight were effective, and three were ineffective. In addition, there were no toxic side reactions as seen with other anticancer drugs, such as arrest of bone marrow, digestive tract reaction, reaction of tunica mucosa oris, and baldness. On the contrary, with current treatment, all the patients in the study group had improvements in spirit, appetite, digestive function, physical strength, and immunologic function of the body. The drugs were also shown effective on hepatitis B, rhinallergosis, pulmonary TB, and coronary heart disease. Therefore, the drugs are notably better than other antitumor drugs.

The essential ingredients of "C" Formula and "Y" Formula, sheep sorrel, burdock root, schidigera yucca and fennel, etc., have distinct anti-inflammatory, analgesic, peptogenic, and repercussive function. The results of this group of observations showed that the combined use of "C" Formula and "Y" Formula had confirmed therapeutic effect on the treatment and prevention of tumor. They could improve the immunologic function of the body and the overall health of the patient. The drugs had no obvious toxic side reaction. (Yan et al. 1996, Discussion)

With the case study comprised of two hundred forty-five cases, it is known that these cases included seventy stomach cancer patients, eighty-five lung cancer patients, and ninety nasopharyngeal cancer (NPC) patients. The study was monitored under the stringent guidance of the Chinese Ministry of Health at the three major hospitals mentioned earlier. It was because of the favorable results of this case study that the import permits for CESSIAC® and YUCCALIVE® (Kang Ji and Yu Kang) were issued by China's Ministry of Health. They are classified as medicine for a Class A disease. (In China, Class A denotes life threatening.)

From 1994 through 1998, Dr. John K. F. Fong, a Chinese MD, served as the chief medical consultant for MPS International in Hong Kong. During those years, he handled thousands of patients in his practice. In 1996, he prepared a clinical summary from 583 cases of patients taking CESSIAC® ("C" Formula) and YUCCALIVE® ("Y" Formula) (Fong, 1996). The cases were selected using diagnosis standards outlined in the Chinese, *Practical Internal Medicine* and the British, *Davidson's Principles and Practice of Medicine.* In the 583 cases, 288 had cancer, 176 had rhinallergosis, 84 had asthma, and 35 had lupus erythematosus. The estimation standards were defined as follows:

Healing: Symptoms disappeared and all examination results resumed to normal.

Notably Effective: Symptoms basically disappeared; and all examination results basically resumed to normal.

Effective: Symptoms remitted to some extent, and all examinations showed some improvements.

Ineffective: None of the symptoms showed any changes, or only some of the symptoms had minor changes. (Fong 1996, Section III)

The patients were administered 60 ml T.I.D. of "C" Formula. It was diluted with the same amount of warm distilled water and taken on an empty stomach. (Warm water aids in absorption.) They received 30 ml Q.D. of "Y" Formula. Dr. Fong summarizes his findings:

Of the 288 cases of cancer, 145 cases were notably effective, accounting for 50.37 percent; 100 cases were effective, accounting for 43.70 percent; (43 were ineffective: 14.93 percent).

The most effective cases were observed on the patients with intestinal cancer, malignant lymphoma, nasopharyngeal carcinoma, and leukemia.

Of the 84 cases of asthma, 11 were healed, 30 were notably effective, 36 were effective, and total effective rate was 92.47 percent.

Of the 176 cases of rhinallergosis, the total effective rate was 94.89 percent.

For the 35 cases of lupus erythematosus, the total effective rate was 92.86. (Fong 1996, Section IX)

The results of these Chinese studies and investigations demonstrate the efficacy of an Essiac formulation (CESSIAC®), in conjunction with a potentiating (enhancing) formulation, (YUCCALIVE®), using the stringent clinical testing standards of the Chinese Ministry of Health. These data support the huge anecdotal evidence already offered. Both of these Chinese cancer medicines are available to those living in the United States and Canada as an herbal remedy. So a very effective cancer remedy is available to us. However, it is somewhat expensive.

Another manufacturer of an Essiac formulation also reports international interest in their product. Flor-Essence, a previously mentioned Essiac-like product manufactured by Flora, discusses ongoing research of their product on their website. They state:

> Research has shown that even those undergoing conventional medical treatments demonstrate many positive results with this tea. A literature review conducted by the University of Texas Center for Alternative Medicine Research (UT-CAM) identified 107 references on the principal herbs used in Flor-Essence. Flora, an herbal manufacturing company, has initiated pre-clinical and clinical evaluations of Flor-Essence in Russia with the Russian Ministry of Health, who are interested in using Flor-Essence to treat victims of Chernobyl.
>
> Pre-clinical trials with several different animal species have documented that Flor-Essence possesses: 1) immuno-stimulatory activity; 2) immuno-modulatory activity; 3) adaptogenic activity; 4) anti-toxic, gastro-protective, hepato-protective, and anti-hypoxic activity; 5) capillary-protective effects, and 6) anti-inflammation that is chemically induced. (Diamond 2003, para. 3)

All of these investigations into the efficacy and merit of Essiac and its prevalence of use demonstrate the ongoing and undying interest in this herbal preparation. Next, the safety of Essiac will be discussed, as well as precautions and contraindications. It will also be compared and contrasted to conventional cancer therapies.

# SAFETY AND
# COST OF ESSIAC VERSUS
# CONVENTIONAL THERAPY

Thus far, it has been clearly demonstrated that Essiac is very safe and non-toxic. This has been proven anecdotally and clinically. Even detractors or skeptics of Essiac have never challenged this. However, any ingested substance can potentially cause an allergic reaction. In addition, many herbs and medications are to be avoided during pregnancy and breast-feeding. Most manufacturers of Essiac caution against its use during pregnancy and breast-feeding.

Brinker (1998), while providing a detailed account of various herb contraindications, does not mention Essiac, but provides some cautions on the individual herbs. Burdock is a hypoglycemic herb, which means that it can lower blood sugar levels, so, insulin dosage in diabetics could be affected. It is speculated that it possesses an oxytocic effect (inducing uterine contraction), so is contraindicated in pregnancy. Slippery Elm Bark and Sheep Sorrel have properties that modify intestinal absorption similar to that of a diet high in fiber. No specific contraindications are noted, just the potential for slowed or altered absorption. In addition, Sheep Sorrel contains oxalate, a substance that is implicated in the formation of some kidney stones. Finally, Turkey Rhubarb is contraindicated in pregnancy. It also has a cathartic (laxative) effect, which may aggravate conditions like irritable bowel syndrome, colitis, Crohn's disease, appendicitis, and hemorrhoids.

Two books on Essiac mention possible side effects from the tea. Olson (1998) mentions:

Though side effects are rare when taking Essiac, there are three general effects:

1. Nausea and/or indigestion, generally caused by eating or drinking too soon before or after drinking the tea
2. Severe intestinal or digestive discomfort, [which is] caused principally because as toxins dissolve, the body tries to eliminate them quickly.
3. An increase in the size of an existing tumor, caused by the metastasized cells gathering at the original site before the tumor softens and reduces in size. (61)

Snow and Klein (1999) describe possible side effects:

Essiac can have some side effects, which might give cause for concern unless they are understood, including:

a. Swelling: occurs when metastasized cells gather into the primary tumor.

b.  Cottage cheese effect: resembling curds and clear liquid, occurs as the cancer breaks up and discharges from either the bodily orifices or from localized cysts or swellings. A jelly-like substance can also be discharged or coughed up from the lungs.

c.  More frequent passing of urine/defecation and other inexplicable discharges occurring as the body detoxifies. If the symptoms are severe, with related nausea and pain, stop taking the formula for a few days until all the symptoms have subsided. When you start drinking it again, take half an ounce every other day, gradually resuming the original dosage. Remember that all diseases have a life cycle and a rhythm of their own, so follow your own judgment according to what your body is telling you about the dosage it needs.

d.  Aching "on site" and headaches, linked to the detoxification process, have been noted as sometimes occurring when taking Essiac after surgery. Treat as for (c) and drink more water to flush out toxins from the body.

e.  Fever or chills: sometimes occurring when the Essiac starts working directly on the cancerous cells. (49-50)

The previously mentioned clinical summary of the 583 patients treated with "C" Formula in China, mentions the following toxic reactions:

During the clinical use of "C" Formula (CESSIAC®), [containing the four original herbs], there were thirty-one cases showing uncomfortable symptoms: temporary decrease of physical strength, hyposthenia (weakness), and eighteen cases showing abdominal distension, constipation, diarrhea, and uncomfortable feeling in the abdomen. No withdrawal of the drugs and special treatments were needed since the toxic reactions remitted spontaneously with continued use of "C" Formula. (Fong 1996, Section VI)

These possible side effects and cautions are mild compared to most pharmaceutical agents. Many over-the-counter drugs list far more extensive or serious side effects on the packaging of their products. For instance, Tylenol® (acetaminophen), a common pain reliever, disclaims that it may cause liver damage. Many prescription drugs advertised on television quickly disclose a laundry list of possible side effects at the end of the commercial, many of which are worse than the ailment they are used to treat.

How do these possible reactions to Essiac compare to those of conventional treatments for cancer? Chemotherapy is one of the primary forms of conventional cancer treatment today, along with surgery and radiation. Paclitaxel is a chemotherapy agent regularly used in the treatment of breast and lung cancers, as well as other types of cancer. It, like many chemotherapy agents, causes a decrease of red blood cells in the patient. It may interfere with menstrual cycles in females and may stop sperm production in males. It cannot be used during pregnancy as it may harm the fetus.

MedlinePlus Drug Information, a service of the US National Library of Science and the National Institutes of Health, lists the following possible side effects for the chemotherapy agent Paclitaxel:

- Nausea and vomiting
- Loss of appetite

- Change in taste
- Thinned or brittle hair
- Pain in the joints of the arms or legs lasting two to three days
- Changes in color of the nails
- Tingling in the hands or toes
- Mouth blistering
- Fatigue
- Unusual bruising or bleeding
- Pain, redness, or swelling at the injection site
- Change in normal bowel habits
- Fever
- Chills
- Cough
- Sore throat
- Difficulty swallowing
- Dizziness
- Shortness of breath
- Severe exhaustion
- Skin rash
- Facial flushing
- Chest pain

(2003a, Side Effects)

In addition, it is mentioned that Paclitaxel must be taken with Decadron (dexamethasone), a corticosteroid drug, which has its own list of nineteen side effects. (MedlinePlus 2003b)

In the case of breast cancer, roughly 25 percent of women diagnosed with the disease have a more aggressive form called HER2 positive breast cancer. For this particular type of cancer, a newer drug is now used to help extend lives. It is called Herceptin (trastuzumab), and it specifically targets the HER2 protein that is over expressed in these types of tumors. Herceptin is a humanized antibody and it is used in conjunction with the chemotherapy drug, paclitaxel (or other chemotherapies), or alone, depending on the patient's prior treatment regimen. MedlinePlus Drug Information lists the following side effects and warnings for Herceptin (trastuzumab):

> IMPORTANT WARNING: Trastuzumab can cause heart damage. Tell your doctor if you are taking cyclophosphamide (Cytoxan, Neosar), daunorubicin (DaunoXome), doxorubicin (Adriamycin, Rubex), or idarubicin (Idamycin) (chemotherapy agents). Keep all appointments with your doctor and the laboratory. Your doctor will order certain lab tests to check your response to trastuzumab. Trastuzumab may cause severe or fatal allergic reactions. Usually this reaction occurs within 24 hours of receiving treatment, but it may occur days after treatment. You should call for help or go to an emergency room immediately if you experience difficulty breathing; swelling of the lips, throat, or inside of you mouth; dizziness or faint-ing; hives; or a severe skin rash. (2003b, Important Warning)

Side effects from trastuzumab are common and usu-ally occur while the drug is being infused. Your doctor may stop your treatment or give you medications to treat these symptoms.

They include:

- Chills or shaking chills
- Nausea
- Vomiting
- Pain at tumor site or in the abdomen or back
- Shortness of breath
- Muscle weakness or stiffness
- Rash
- Headache

If the following side effects occur after infusion, this should be reported to the doctor:

- Loss of appetite
- Diarrhea
- Sleeplessness
- Runny nose
- Sore throat
- Sinus pain
- Headache
- Fatigue
- Abdominal pain
- Unusual bruising or bleeding
- Swelling of the feet or ankles
- Rapid heartbeat
- Difficulty breathing
- Wheezing while sleeping
- Fever
- Upper respiratory tract infection
- Chills or shaking chills
- Excessive coughing

(2003c, Side Effects)

The possible side effects from taking the three above-mentioned drugs (Paclitaxel, Decadron and Herceptin) seem staggering when viewed this way. Further, consider that oncologists routinely prescribe anti-nausea medications, antihistamines, and pain-relievers to cancer sufferers in addition to the primary therapy to help ease symptoms caused by the disease and the treatments. These, of course, are not without their side effects. So, cancer patients must risk numerous possible side effects in the hopes of extending their lives.

Genentech, the manufacturer of Herceptin, published the results of randomized, controlled clinical trials on the safety and efficacy of this drug (2005a). In one study, 469 patients participated. They all had metastatic breast cancer and they had not been previously treated with chemotherapy for metastatic disease. The patients were randomly grouped so that some received chemotherapy alone, and some received chemotherapy in addition to Herceptin. The test measured time of progression, overall response rate, median duration of response, and median survival time. The group receiving Herceptin and chemotherapy had more favorable results than those taking chemotherapy alone. Genentech (2005a) reports the following results from a Phase III clinical trial:

**Median Survival Time (in months)**
All Chemotherapy (234 patients) . . . . . . . . . . . . . . . . . . . 20.3
Herceptin + Chemotherapy (235 patients) . . . . . . . . . . . 25.1
(Table 1)

Genentech (2005a) also reported statistics compiled regarding Herceptin's cardiotoxicity:

**Percentage of Patients with Cardiac Dysfunction**

Herceptin Alone (213 patients) . . . . . . . . . . . . . . . . . . . . . . .7%

Herceptin + Paclitaxel (91 patients) . . . . . . . . . . . . . . . . . . 11%

Paclitaxel Alone (95 patients) . . . . . . . . . . . . . . . . . . . . . . . .1%

Herceptin + Anthracycline + Cyclophosphamide
(143 patients). . . . . . . . . . . . . . . . . . . . . . . . . . . . . . . . . . .28%

Anthracylcine = Cyclophosphamide Alone (135 patients) . . .7%
(Table 3)

Harrar gives an upbeat account of improved outcomes for breast cancer patients taking Herceptin, but closes with, "However, up to 16 percent of women in these trials developed congestive heart failure, so patients older than age fifty or those with heart risks should discuss the pros and cons with their doctors. And your co-pay could be sizable. A year's worth of treatment costs about $47,000" (2006, 40).

One more example of a conventional cancer therapy is Avastin (bevacizumab), a drug considered a valuable tool in the treatment of colon cancer. Avastin is also manufactured by Genentech, and efforts to have it used in the treatment of breast and lung cancer are under way. Avastin inhibits the development of new blood vessels that carry vital nutrients to tumors. This process of the development of new blood cells is called angiogenesis. (Shark cartilage is an alternative cancer therapy that is said to work on this premise.)

However, Genentech (2005b) wrote a letter to health-care providers warning them of the danger of strokes and heart attacks in patients treated with Avastin whether done so alone or in combination with chemotherapy. In addition, the list of side effects and the cost of this drug are even more impressive than those of Herceptin. MedlinePlus Drug

Information lists the more common side effects of Avastin (most of which are to be reported to the doctor immediately):

Black, tarry stools; bleeding gums; body aches or pain; chest pain; chills; cloudy urine; cough; cracks in the skin; convulsions; decreased urine output; dilated neck veins; ear congestion; extreme fatigue; fever; high blood pressure; irregular breathing; irregular heartbeat; loss of appetite; loss of heat from the body; lack or loss of strength; loss of voice; mood changes; nasal congestion; pain; painful or difficult urination; pinpoint red spots on the skin; redness; runny nose; shortness of breath; sore throat; sores, ulcers, or white spots on lips or in mouth; swollen glands; swelling of the face, fingers, feet, or lower legs; troubled breathing; tightness in chest; unusual bleeding or bruising; unusual tiredness or weakness; vomiting of blood or material that looks like coffee grounds; watery or bloody diarrhea; weight gain; wheezing; yellow skin; belching; bloody nose; change in walking or balance; clumsiness or unsteadiness; excess flow of tears; hair loss; thinning of hair; heartburn; indigestion; low blood pressure; weight loss.

Less common are difficulty having a bowel movement (stool); fainting; stomach tenderness.

Rare are blisters, coma; confusion; convulsions; decreased urine output, increased thirst, muscle pain or cramps; open sores; pale skin. (2005d, Side Effects of This Medicine)

Genentech, the manufacturer of Avastin, also published results of this drug's efficacy (2005b). It compared cancer patients who were treated with a standard therapy for colon and rectal cancer, IFL (irinotecan/ fluorouracil/leucovorin), to patients who were treated with Avastin, in addition to IFL. The overall survival rates follow:

IFL + Placebo (411 patients) . . . . . . . . . . . . . . . . . .15.6 months (median)

IFL + Avastin (402 patients) . . . . . . . . . . . . . . . . . . . 20.3 months (median)

(2005b, Table 1)

*The New York Times* recently reported that Avastin, customarily used in the treatment of colon cancer, might now be used to treat other cancers like those of the breasts and lungs:

Doctors say they are excited about the prospect of Avastin, a drug already widely used for colon cancer, as a crucial new treatment for breast and lung cancer, too. But doctors are also cringing at the price the maker, Genentech, plans to charge for it: about $100,000 a year. (Berenson 2006, para. 1)

The comparison of Essiac therapies to these conventional cancer treatments reveals striking and alarming differences.

Essiac's efficacy has been extensively documented anecdotally, suggested by research done on the tea and its components, and proven by quality clinical studies conducted under the supervision of the Chinese Ministry of Health. It has demonstrated favorable outcomes while also improving the patients' well-being and quality of life. Further, it is non-toxic, has minimal possible side effects, and it is reasonably priced.

The cost of Essiac products in the United States and Canada vary depending on manufacturer, dosage, and whether the preparation is purchased as a pre-brewed tea or as dry herbs to be brewed by the purchaser. The dry herbs range in price from $2.00 to $25.00 per ounce. One ounce of dried herbs typically yields thirty ounces of liquid. A pre-brewed thirty-two-ounce bottle of tea costs between $16.00 and $40.00. The dosage of tea is between one and six ounces per day, depending on the reason for taking the tea. For example, a person who takes the tea as a tonic or cancer preventative may take one ounce per day, whereas, a person with advanced cancer may take six ounces per day. Therefore, if a person brewed one thirty-two-ounce bottle (using $2.00 per ounce dry herbs), his cost per year would be roughly $24.00 if he took one ounce per day. Conversely, if someone purchased the pre-brewed tea at $40.00 per bottle and took six ounces per day—2,190 ounces, or roughly sixty-eight bottles per year—his cost would be $2,720 annually.

Alternately, the conventional drug therapies mentioned, which are considered cutting edge and promising, in reality offer clinical proof of extending a cancer patient's life by only months. These are months lived with the possibility of debilitating side effects from the treatment, and their prohibitive costs leave them unavailable to many.

Most cancer patients are totally unaware of these grim statistics. Doctors and pharmaceutical manufacturers present these modest gains in lifespan more positively to them. They may claim that a drug increases survival by one third, leading the patient to believe that one-third more people will survive their disease by using it. But in reality, this means that if a cancer patient is expected to survive for only nine months, the addition of this drug therapy will extend their survival time to twelve months. One might wonder how many cancer patients would agree to the suffering these therapies often cause if they were privy to all this information up front.

Consider the following opinions held by those who are most familiar with this information. William Campbell Douglass ll, MD, a renowned physician and author of many books on health, writes:

> To understand the utter hypocrisy of chemotherapy, consider the following: The McGill Cancer Center in Canada, one of the largest and most prestigious cancer treatment centers in the world, did a study of oncologists to determine how they would respond to a diagnosis of cancer. On the confidential questionnaire, fifty-eight out of sixty-four doctors said that all chemotherapy programs were unacceptable to them and their family members.
>
> The overriding reason for this decision was that the drugs are ineffective and have an unacceptable degree of toxicity. These are the same doctors who will tell you that their chemotherapy treatments will shrink your tumor and prolong your life! (2002, para. 1)

With the state of current cancer treatments, what options do cancer sufferers have? Patients that do their research and question their doctors are often dismissed. Many doctors suggest that alternative therapies are dangerous, or at best worthless, and they frighten their patients about using them. This can create an agonizing situation for a cancer sufferer, who often feels helpless in his fate. He can choose a conventional therapy that involves poisoning himself and/or disabling his already impaired immune system to kill cancer cells, or he can choose an "unproven" therapy that seeks to heal his immune system and allow it to eliminate the cancer by itself. But by choosing the latter, he lives in fear that he may be signing his own death warrant, as many oncologists would lead him to believe.

This is not to suggest that the conventional and the alternative have to be mutually exclusive. It has already been demonstrated that Essiac alleviates many of the undesirable effects of chemotherapy and radiation, but that may not be all. Balch (2002) lists findings that support that the use of Essiac may make standard chemotherapy more effective. She states:

> Essiac's efficacy against cancer can be explained in part by the cancer-fighting characteristics of herbs in the formula. Two chemicals in rhubarb, emodin and rhein, may stop the growth of melanoma, breast cancers, and hepatic carcinoma. One of these chemicals, emodin, has been found in the laboratory to greatly enhance the effects of conventional chemotherapies. It makes breast cancer cells more sensitive to paclitaxol (Taxol) and makes certain types of lung cancer cells more sensitive to cisplatin (Platinol) and doxorubicin (Adriamycin, Rubex). A closely related chemical, aloe emodin, found in sheep sorrel, has significant activity against leukemia cells. (2002, 155)

Perhaps Essiac and other alternative treatments would be viewed more positively by Western medical practitioners if they would consider them as potential adjunct therapies.

Since there is evidence that Essiac alleviates the negative side effects of traditional treatment and possibly enhances its desired effects, it follows that more investigation is warranted.

This scrutiny of Essiac products and their conventional counterparts helps to shed light on a growing phenomenon evolving in cancer treatment. There has been little significant achievement in the war on cancer during the last century. Some small battles have been won, but the war rages on despite a gargantuan expenditure of human suffering and financial investment. Patient dissatisfaction with the state of cancer medicine today is leading huge numbers to seek out complementary/alternative medicine (CAM). These patients want to expand their treatment options, hoping to enhance their clinical outcomes. In other words, CAM offers them hope. The prevalence of use, nature of, and reason for CAM modalities will be discussed in the next section.

# COMPLEMENTARY/ ALTERNATIVE MEDICINE (CAM) THERAPIES

Therapies other than those traditionally taught in the medical schools of the United States, Canada, and Britain, are generally classified as alternative medicine. These include chiropractic, naturopathy, homeopathy, faith healing, traditional Chinese medicine (TCM), and Ayurveda (traditional Indian medicine). Some forms of alternative medicine are more prone to be classified as complementary medicine. That is, they are more likely to be utilized or condoned by mainstream or traditional practitioners (MDs). These are modalities like acupuncture, massage, biofeedback, meditation, yoga, and nutritional therapies. Essiac and other herbals such as curcumin, echinacea, grape seed extract, Hoxsey, and milk thistle are all examples of alternative cancer therapies.

One might make the case that the conventional medicine of today is really the alternative—the new kid on the block. In the grand scheme of things, many CAM modalities have stood the test of time, with many being used for centuries and some, like acupuncture, for thousands of years. It would seem that these would be more aptly referred to as traditional. One criticism of Western medicine by other cultures is that it is somewhat arrogant in its dismissal of or indifference to the healing wisdom of the ages.

Another difference between mainstream Western medicine and alternative therapies is the approach to dealing with disease. Western medicine is strong diagnostically, but deals with disease primarily with pharmaceutical agents and surgery. Control or elimination of symptoms is its main objective. It is highly specialized, with physicians treating particular body systems. Further, it puts less emphasis on preventative strategies and more on aggressive suppression of symptoms after the disease process has already been initiated (immunization being the exception).

CAM modalities, on the other hand, tend to be more holistic, looking at the patient as a whole. The patient's emotional, spiritual, and physical well-being is of primary concern, as well as his or her environment. Although, some CAM therapies treat symptoms, many are meant to boost the immune system so that the body can heal itself.

Many patients first investigate complementary/alternative medicine when they feel that their current medical care is failing them or insufficient in some way. Often word of mouth leads them to CAM. Whatever the reason, CAM use increases every year. There are dozens of references and studies published on the prevalence of and reason for alternative therapy use. Some of these will be mentioned to qualify and quantify this growing phenomenon.

MedlinePlus reports the following statistic: "Despite the lack of available scientific evidence, Essiac and Essiac-like products (with similar ingredients) remain popular among patients, particularly in those with cancer. Essiac is most commonly taken as a tea. A survey conducted in the year 2000 found almost 15 percent of Canadian women with breast cancer to be using Essiac" (2005e, para. 5).

Another large study of Flor-Essence® users conducted by the University of Texas in 2000 reported that of 1,577 cancer (breast, lung, and prostate) patients, 50.6 percent experienced improvement of symptoms while taking the tea, with 6.6 percent reporting adverse events. Approximately 85 percent of these had been treated previously by conventional means, and 37 percent were being treated simultaneously with the tea and conventional therapy. Nearly two thirds of the respondents discussed using Essiac with their physicians. The study concluded, "The tonic is widely distributed. Many cancer patients combine conventional treatment with the tonic and attribute benefits to the tonic. The use of herbal formulas is a public health issue; thus, assessment of clinical benefit and potential interaction with cancer treatment is warranted" (Richardson et al. 2000, Abstract).

Another study published in the *Journal of Clinical Oncology* sought to determine the prevalence of CAM use by breast cancer survivors. Boon et al. (2000) used a questionnaire format and found that two thirds of the respondents reported using CAM—most with the intention of boosting their immune systems. The most commonly used CAM products were vitamins/minerals, herbal medicines, green tea, special foods, and Essiac. Nearly half of the respondents had informed their doctors of their CAM use. The study concluded, "CAM use is common among Canadian breast cancer survivors, many of whom are discussing CAM therapy options with their physicians. Knowledge of CAM therapies is necessary for physicians and other health care practitioners to help patients make informed choices. CAM use may play a role in the positive benefits associated with support group attendance" (Boon et al. 2000, 2515).

A survey performed by the National Institutes of Health in Bethesda, MD, sought to describe CAM use by adult cancer patients enrolled in the National Cancer Institute (NCI) clinical trials. The study was published in the *Oncology Nurse Forum*, and it utilized a ninety-nine-item questionnaire. It found that 63 percent of respondents used at least one form of CAM, but the average was two forms of CAM therapy. These therapies included nutritional supplementation, relaxation, diet (macrobiotic, vegetarian), imagery, and exercise. Most reported using CAM to relieve the discomfort of treatment, stress, anxiety, fatigue, and to gain more control of their lives. One hundred percent of the respondents believed that their quality of life was improved by CAM use. The report concluded, "Patients with cancer use various complementary therapies to cope with their disease and the rigors of clinical trials. Women and those with higher educational backgrounds were more frequent users" (Sparber et al. 2000, 623).

Another study of CAM use and prevalence was conducted by the College of Nursing at the University of South Florida.

The survey participants consisted of one hundred five breast cancer patients. The study found that 64 percent of the participants regularly used vitamin/mineral supplementation, and 33 percent regularly used antioxidants, herbs, and health foods. Stress reduction techniques were also employed, with 49 percent using prayer and other spiritual healing, 37 percent belonging to support groups, and 21 percent using humor therapy. The study noted, "More frequent CAM use was observed among study participants who had undergone previous chemotherapy treatment and those with more than a high school education. Also, being less satisfied with their primary physician was associated with patients' more frequent CAM use" (Lengacher et al. 2002, 1445).

A study of CAM use was also conducted by the School of Health and Social Services at the University of Wales Institute-Cardiff in the UK. It, too, looked at prevalence of use, but also was concerned with the level of satisfaction CAM users felt. In their survey of 1,697 cancer patients, 49.6 percent reported using at least one CAM therapy. These included over-the-counter diets, supplements, and remedies. The study noted, "Dissatisfaction with CAM use was low, and most users indicated that they represented value for the money" (Harris et al. 2003, 249).

Another study regarding CAM use was conducted by the National Foundation for Alternative Medicine, Washington, DC, which looked at the discrepant views of cancer patients and oncologists. The study's objective was to determine how their views differed and to understand the reason for failure to disclose CAM use by many patients. The patients who did not disclose their CAM use reported that their reasons for keeping quiet were due to uncertainty of its benefits, and because their oncologists had not asked them about it. Physicians believed that patients did not disclose CAM use because they thought it unimportant, and that the doctor might disapprove or try to discourage them, or even discontinue treating them.

The physicians felt that patients sought out CAM therapies because they are nontoxic, but also because CAM therapies offered them hope and helped them feel some measure of control over an incurable disease. Patients were more likely to say they sought out CAM therapies to improve immunity and quality of life. Both patients and oncologists agreed that CAM modalities could offer relief of symptoms and side effects of conventional treatment. The report concluded, "Oncologists and cancer patients hold discrepant views on CAM that may contribute to a communication gap. Nevertheless, physicians should ask patients about CAM use, discuss the possible benefits, and advise of potential risks" (Richardson et al. 2004, 797).

Finally, a study was done by the Division of Medical Oncology, Department of Medicine, at the Mayo Foundation and Mayo Clinic College of Medicine in Rochester, MN. This involved a survey of patients with advanced malignancies who were enrolled in phase I chemotherapy trials. Of the respondents, 88.2 percent used at least one form of CAM therapy. Of these CAM users, 89.3 percent used vitamin and mineral preparations, 29.8 percent used green tea, 13.1 percent used Echinacea, and 9.5 percent used Essiac. The most popular non-pharmacologic CAM therapies used were prayer and spiritual practices, which were used by 52.1 percent. The study's conclusion states, "CAM use is common among patients in phase I trials and should be ascertained by investigators, because some of the agents used may interact with investigational agents and affect adverse effects and/or efficacy" (Dy et al. 2004, 4810). It is of interest to note that in this study, the conclusion recommends that CAM use be monitored in order to identify possible negative interactions, but not positive ones.

In summary, these studies illustrate the growing trend of CAM use by cancer patients. (CAM modalities are utilized by many individuals for various health reasons, but for the purpose of this discussion, only those studies involving cancer survivors were examined.) There is increasing use of complementary/alternative medicine for many reasons. Patients believe that their lives are improved and they report satisfaction with CAM modalities. They believe these therapies improve immunity, help alleviate the side effects of conventional treatment, and reduce stress, anxiety, and depression.

It is noted that women are more likely to utilize CAM therapies than men are, as are those with higher educational backgrounds. Patients who have received prior chemotherapy are also more likely to try CAM, as are those who report dissatisfaction with their doctors and/or the standard cancer treatments they've been given.

It is interesting to note that doctors and their patients have discrepant views on CAM therapies, and that many patients do not inform their doctors of their CAM use. The studies all conclude that because of the prevalence of use, CAM therapies need further evaluation. Clinical assessment is warranted for the safety and well-being of patients. This evaluation can validate the worth of CAM modalities or identify potential problems. Because many cancer patients use conventional and complementary/alternative medicine simultaneously, it is imperative that the effects of this combined use be studied carefully.

# CASE DESCRIPTIONS AND PATIENT TESTIMONIALS

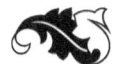

The prolific use of Essiac tea is a testament to the power of "word of mouth" and personal testimony. Shared experiences have educated and benefited man throughout the ages. Those who advertise Essiac are really the users themselves. This is why the belief in Essiac's value has never ceased, and, in fact, has grown consistently over the last ninety years. Those who suffer from cancer and those who care for them spread the word in the hopes of alleviating the suffering of others.

As stated before, allopathic medicine is reluctant to place much worth in anecdotal evidence with regard to non-conventional treatments. When positive results occur, they are often attributed to the placebo effect. That is, the patient's condition improves during treatment, but the specific treatment used cannot be considered the cause of the improvement. Put another way, the patient believes so strongly that she will benefit from the treatment that this belief is the reason for any improvement.

There is a certain amount of irony here. Medical practitioners are reluctant to acknowledge a patient's testimony when it concerns an alternative treatment, yet they rely heavily on what a patient communicates to them when making diagnoses and prescribing for them. Is a patient's word only reliable within the realm of conventional medicine? Is the placebo effect more likely to occur when using an alternative treatment than any other treatment? These questions warrant consideration.

At this point, some case histories and personal testimonies from physicians and patients, beyond those previously included in the history portion, will be presented. They illustrate the reason for Essiac use.

> Glum (1988) opens his chronicle of Essiac with the following passage:
>
> On October 5, 1983, E. Bruce Hendrick, the chief of neurosurgery at the University of Toronto's Hospital for Sick Children, wrote to the Canadian Minister of Health and Welfare saying that Dr. Hendrick supported a scientific clinical trial of the cancer treatment compound known as "Essiac."
>
> Dr. Hendrick stated that after they started on Essiac, eight of ten patients with surgically treated tumors of the central nervous system had "escaped from the conventional methods of therapy including both radiation and chemotherapy."
>
> Dr. Hendrick wrote that he was "most impressed with the effectiveness of the treatment and its lack

of side effects." He closed with this: "I feel that this method of treatment should be given serious consideration and would benefit from a scientific clinical trial."

With that letter, Dr. Hendrick joined a long list of physicians dating back more than sixty years who have spoken in favor of Essiac as a cancer treatment. (1988, i)

Fong (1996) reports some typical cases from the 583 cases of patients treated with CESSIAC® (Formula C) and YUCCALIVE® (Formula Y) in Hong Kong. (Recall from the section on Essiac's efficacy that CESSIAC® is an Essiac formulation and that YUCCALIVE® is a potentiating herbal tea that enhances the action of CESSIAC®). Two of the cancer cases follow:

Dequm Yao, female, fifty-one years old. On April 1, 1994, the patient underwent an intestinal cancer removal operation at Nadasu Hospital of Hong Kong. After the operation, the patient was treated with chemotherapy. Without any improvement, the patient still had the following symptoms: asthenia [weakness], hyphema [hemorrhage in the anterior chamber of the eye], lassitude [fatigue], hematochezia [passage of blood in the feces]. When the patient was re-hospitalized on March 20, 1994, it was found that the tumor had transferred to the liver, and an operation was needed. When the patient was hesitating, her younger sister recommended Formula C and Formula Y to her. Upon drinking the teas, within a couple of days, the following appeared: (1) Secretion from nasal cavity was increased and black ball shaped substances were spitted out; (2) Large amount of black watery feces were defecated, and the spirit and appetite improved. With the continued use of the teas, the magnetic resonance scan on May 10 found that the two shadows in the liver had disappeared, and the doctor considered that an operation was no longer needed. The patient was required to be reexamined after three months.

Shuhua Li, female, forty-eight years old. The patient was diagnosed to have lymph node cancer on the left neck at Sha Tin Prince of Wales Hospital in Hong Kong in September 1993. In October, the patient underwent a cancer removal operation followed by radiation therapy. Without any improvement, the cancer was found on April 13, 1994 to have transferred to the supraclavicular lymph nodes on the right side of the neck with a size of about 4 cm. With the recommendation of a friend, the patient started drinking Formula C and Formula Y on April 22. On June 2 (after drinking the teas for over a month), the enlarged lymph nodes had reduced to 0.5 cm. On June 28, the tumor had disappeared. (1996, Section VII).

Thomas (1993) provides copies of testimonial letters written by cancer patients or their loved ones chronicling their use of Essiac as a treatment. Two of these letters follow:

I am writing in regards to the "Flor-Essence" herbal product and how it has turned my mother's health around.

In November 1991, my mother (Elsie Gaspard) was diagnosed with cancer of the throat and stomach and given three months to live. On Boxing Day, my sister Vi heard about your herbal tea (Flor-Essence) from her friend. She purchased some from you, brewed it up, and made it available to Mom through the rest of the family. Mom was in bad shape; the doctor said she was too far gone for chemotherapy and prescribed morphine for the pain. He said, "Just try to keep her comfortable— that is all that can be done." Nobody was very enthusiastic about the herbal tea; therefore, she didn't receive it on a regular basis, and she threw up much of that. She was thin as a rail and her eyes were dark sunken circles. She seemed oblivious of everything.

On May 16, an article on "Flor-Essence" came out in the Vancouver Sun. There were several encouraging accounts on how the medicine had amazing results with other cancer patients. Our family became greatly enthusiastic about the medicine. My sister Barbara visited Mom for a while to see that she took the tea on a regular basis. As a result, Mom's health improved dramatically through the months. She gained weight; her appetite and mental capabilities came back.

Best of all, her doctor diagnosed her almost cancer free on or about October 1, 1992.

Thank you, sincerely, William Gaspard

\*\*\*

In March of 1994, my mother after a few months of not being able to walk, phoned me in Vancouver to take her to the doctor. "Come quickly," she said. "I think I'm dying." The doctor diagnosed breast cancer, which had spread to the bones. He was angry she had not gone for a check-up earlier. Now it was too late, he said. Maybe with chemo and radiation she might last for two years at the most, but he thought probably six months, considering how far the cancer had spread. It was in her hips, spine, shoulders, and base of [the] skull. When the shock of all this wore off a little, I went into action, determined to do everything I possibly could to at least ease her pain. I remember praying very hard and asking God to show me what to do. That same day I received five calls from concerned friends all telling me about this Essiac tea. This was the message. That same day I went out and got the tea and all available information on it.

I started her on the tea morning and night and never forgot to give it to her. After a few months, I was beginning to lose hope, as she was getting much worse. She was very ill, full of pain, couldn't eat or go to the bathroom; she looked like a skeleton held together by her skin. At this point, the doctor said she probably wouldn't last two weeks. This was at the beginning of August 1994. At the end of August, something happened—her appetite returned, and she started walking, slowly at first because she had been in bed for sixth months. Her pain was gone and her energy returned. Slowly she built her strength, gained weight, and started doing more things she hadn't done in a long time. This was a miracle.

Today, my mom has an active life, many friends, lives on her own in Kelowna, and is looking forward to the birth of a new grandchild in September 1995. The doctors seemed very shocked and could offer no explanation. I'm convinced that what really helped her was the Flor-Essence tea I consistently made her drink.

The greatest benefit of this was the easing of her great pain. For this, I thank God for having led me to this tea, which I had never heard of before.

Thank you, Anna Todesco (Appendix)

Percival (1994) provides numerous testimonials as to the benefits of Essiac for many conditions. Here is one cancer patient's story:

Our family was devastated when my mother-in-law, Myrna, informed us that she had been diagnosed with cancer. In her case, it was ovarian cancer that had spread to the lymph glands and then into the lungs. It was diagnosed as inoperative, and the doctors told her to get her affairs in order. After a hysterectomy, they said, she would have about six months to live. The tumors in her lungs were too numerous to remove. My sister-in-law asked if there was some nutritional approach that might slow the progress of the disease. The doctor assured her there was none. But I nevertheless began to search for alternative remedies. By chance, my father heard a radio program where Essiac was explained.

The remedy was so simple and straightforward that I knew my mother-in-law could take it. She took a little each night. We held our breaths. The doctor and our nurse cousin told us not to get our hopes up. Yet, the weekly X-rays began indicating something they did not expect. Little by little, the tumors in her lungs stabilized, and they began to diminish. The nursing staff at the doctor's office reacted in awe as week after week, the tumors were disappearing, and her blood count returned to normal.

A little more than a year after beginning Essiac, the doctor called to tell Myrna that she was an official miracle. Her charts showed no indication of cancer in any system. To date, five years later, there has been no recurrence of cancer.

J. R. Kirkland, Washington (1994, 20)

Vaughan (2003) compiled the stories of fifty recovered cancer patients. They all describe their often-miraculous recoveries, and are not hesitant to state what they attribute them to. One patient, John Lallo, was diagnosed with a brain tumor. He decided to reject chemotherapy and radiation, which his doctor told him might give him only a year to live. Instead, he took Essiac every day, used oxygen therapy, and made dietary changes like avoiding white flour, sugar, and meat. In his words, "I decided not to fry my brains, and the doctor is shocked I'm still alive. I have had two MRIs, and there has been no cancer so far growing back" (Vaughan 2003, 112).

Another man, Fred Robertson, was diagnosed with prostate cancer, and he credits his recovery to Essiac, a positive attitude, and a devoted spiritual life. He states, "I know that Essiac is the main reason that I have felt so good for the last six years. Not only have I reached remission, but [my] life [today is] better than [it was] throughout my [earlier years]. My oncologist told me, after the sixteen months of Essiac treatment, that I was in remission from a rare blood disorder that I had needed monthly treatments for since 1973. Can it be anything else? Doubtful" (Vaughan 2003, 146).

These are just a small representation of the many testimonials and accounts that can be found on Essiac use. All of the above were published in books, but the Internet is filled with patient testimonials posted by Essiac marketers whose products have benefited many people. Essiac marketers are not permitted to make medical claims about their products, but nothing prevents their customers from telling their stories.

In the interest of further research and personal health, this researcher purchased a pre-brewed Essiac formulation manufactured by Tehachapi Tea Company. I have had rheumatoid arthritis for twenty years, and through this investigation, I learned that many with my condition claim to have been helped by Essiac. I selected the Tehachapi Tea Company on the basis of a recommendation by an independent organization that reviewed numerous products. Also, the company's founder is an RN who has been brewing Essiac since 1996. Only organic herbs are used, and the cost is reasonable, so it is accessible to most people. After taking the product for two weeks, I noticed decreased pain and increased energy. I continue to take it daily, and when I missed taking it for ten days while on vacation, I noticed an exacerbation of my symptoms.

To expand on this research, I contacted Chris Corpening, RN BSN, the company's owner, and told her of my Essiac research; I asked her if she would distribute a research questionnaire for me. She agreed, and was provided with twenty-five questionnaires along with letters of explanation and self-addressed stamped envelopes to be enclosed with orders of their Essiac product, A Nurse's Herbal Tea.

The results of the returned surveys were very much in keeping with the material that has been presented previously.

Some of the statistical results and respondent comments follow:

Six of the twenty-five surveys were returned, representing a 24 percent response rate, with half of the respondents being women and half men. Of the six respondents, four (67 percent) learned about Essiac from others (friends or family), and two (33 percent) from Internet research. Five of the six (83 percent) used it in the treatment of cancer, with one (16 percent) using it to maintain immune system health. The types of cancer being treated were renal cell carcinoma (stage III), lung cancer (stage IV), pancreatic cancer, breast cancer, and one unspecified cancer.

The duration of Essiac usage ranged from nine months to eight years. Four (67 percent) of the respondents listed specific benefits. One (16 percent) listed no specific benefits, but commented that there had been no recurrence of cancer in the two years following a lumpectomy and radiation for breast cancer. She had been taking the herbal tea for a year and a half at the time of the survey. One (16 percent) respondent did not answer the question. Fifty percent of the respondents knew of others who had benefited from Essiac use and all (100 percent) purchased the product pre-brewed, as opposed to buying the dried herbs and brewing their own at a lesser cost. Fifty percent of the tea users did not inform their doctors that they were using it. Thirty-three percent told their doctors about it, and one person did not respond to the question. Some of the respondents' stories and comments follow.

A seventy-four year old female from New York State who wished to remain anonymous returned the questionnaire. Her daughter filled it out for her since her mother does not speak

English. Her mother was diagnosed with pancreatic cancer in 2003, and she received seven months of chemotherapy and six weeks of radiation. The daughter stated that her mother's doctors were aware of her mother's tea use "but they don't really say much." At the time of the survey, her mother had been taking the tea for two years, and when asked what benefits were seen from taking the tea, she replied, "So far, so good!"

A seventy-one-year-old male from Oklahoma, made the following comments: "I use it to maintain my immune system. I have used it for approximately eight years (taking) 2 ounces per day, diluted with 2 ounces of distilled water. I think it keeps my immune system in good shape. I seldom have a cold or any other ailment."

An eighty-year-old man from Tempe, Arizona, was diagnosed with stage IV lung cancer in August of 2000. He said the cancer was "too spread out for radiology or surgery, [so I was] put on chemo treatment once a week." He stated that he continued chemotherapy until September of 2002. When asked if his doctor was aware of his tea use, he responded, "Yes—Dr. said to keep doing it; he had no objections." He has been taking Essiac "since May 2001, started with Flor-essence and switched to Nurse's Tea later, 2 ounces with water at breakfast and bedtime. I have been in stable remission since November 2003. Chest X-ray is clear as of October 24, 2005."

An RN MSN, is a fifty-four year old female from Ohio. She was diagnosed with stage III renal cell carcinoma in April 2005. She had a radical nephrectomy and adrenal removed along with the tumor. She started taking the tea immediately after her discharge from the hospital. When asked if her doctor was aware of her tea use, she replied, "The oncologist is extremely negative, and I tell him nothing (in reference) to alternative therapy." When asked about benefits, she stated, "Three CAT scans all clean for cancer and the doctor is amazed: 'I don't understand why you are doing so well,' After surgery, my doctor kept telling me the cancer would spread, but *every* CAT scan was clear. He has not had to do any treatments beyond [sending me to an] awesome surgeon who got all of the tumor and cancer." This questionnaire was filled out in October 2005. I followed up with an email to her in March 2006, and she continues to be cancer free and doing great.

These cases and testimonials demonstrate the power of shared human experience. They also provide insight into the value of anecdotal evidence as a necessary component of thorough medical research. When conventional medicine fails, patients often become empowered to do their own research. Alternative medicine offers them another avenue of hope.

At this point in the discussion, one might wonder why Essiac has not been investigated thoroughly. The evidence of its value is compelling, to say the least. Its longevity and ever-increasing prevalence of use are impressive. It is safe and cost-effective. Some possible reasons will be explored in the next section.

# REASONS FOR THE LACK OF CLINICAL INVESTIGATION OF ESSIAC

G iven the history and evidence presented thus far, it seems unfathomable that this herbal remedy is largely being ignored by allopathic medicine. What possible reasons would health entities and professionals have for their indifference to something that their patients seek out, research, and purchase on their own in ever-increasing numbers?

Do those providing cancer services feel that the treatment options currently available are of such a high caliber that there is no need for improvement? Are the outcomes of conventional treatment so favorable that alternatives are dismissed as unnecessary? If so, why then does a diagnosis of cancer elicit such terror in those who are stricken and so much concern by those who care about them? The answers to these questions are unfortunate to say the least.

Consider the opinion offered by Andrew Weil, MD, on current cancer therapies. Dr. Weil is a renowned physician and author of many books. He is a graduate of Harvard Medical School, and currently is the Director of the Program in Integrative Medicine at the University of Arizona, Tucson. He is a practitioner of natural and preventive medicine. Weil (1995) writes:

> Current therapies for cancer, both conventional and alternative, are far from satisfactory. Conventional medicine has three main treatments: surgery, radiation, and chemotherapy, of which only the first makes sense. If cancer is in one location only and accessible to a surgeon's knife, it can be excised and eliminated permanently. Unfortunately, only a small percentage of cancers meet those criteria, principally, cancers of the skin and uterine cervix. In far too many cases, cancer has already spread to more than one site by the time of its discovery or is somewhere in the body that is beyond the reach of a surgical cure.
>
> Radiation and chemotherapy are crude treatments that will be obsolete before long. Both work by killing dividing cells; the assumption made by doctors who use them is that cancerous cells divide faster than normal ones. Unfortunately, that is true only for a small percentage of cancers, principally childhood cancers, leukemias, lymphomas, testicular cancer, and a few others. In most cases, cells of cancers have lower division rates than the most active normal tissues of the body; the

skin, the lining of the intestinal tract, the bone marrow, and other immune structures. The well-known side effects of radiation and chemotherapy—hair loss, loss of appetite, nausea, and vomiting—represent damage to the skin and GI tract. Damage to the immune system is less obvious and much more of a concern. If you have cancer and are faced with a decision about whether to use conventional therapies, the question you must try to answer is this: Will the damage done to the cancer justify the damage done to the immune system? (268-269)

Ralph W. Moss, PhD, prolific author and critic of what he refers to as "the cancer establishment," was formerly a science writer and assistant director of public affairs at Memorial Sloan-Kettering Cancer Center. He states that he was "fired in 1977 for opposing the cover-up of positive data on the drug laetrile.... I had, in the words of the *New York Times*, acted in a manner that conflicted with my 'most basic job responsibilities.' In other words, I refused to collaborate in falsifying data" (2002, VII). Since that time, he has written eleven books and created three documentaries concerning cancer related topics. He shares Dr. Weil's assessment of the state of cancer therapy today, but he is much more vocal about the inefficiency and economic motives of the entities that are the driving forces of the cancer industry, namely The Food and Drug Administration, The National Cancer Institute, The American Cancer Society, Memorial Sloan Kettering, and the pharmaceutical drug industry. He writes:

The year 1996 marks the twenty-fifth anniversary of President Nixon's "war on cancer." During this time, the federal government has spent over $25 billion on cancer research, while the American Cancer Society (ACS) and various other private organizations have spent a nearly equal sum. When this war was launched in 1971, leading scientists promised Congress a cure in time for the Bicentennial. That didn't happen, and almost everyone agrees that overall the results of the war on cancer have been meager. (Moss 2002, VII)

Statistics published by the American Cancer Society (ACS) (2006) report the cost of cancer in 2004 at $189.8 billion. Despite this gargantuan expenditure, only modest gains have been made. For example, in 1997, the estimated number of new cancer cases was 1,382,400 and the estimated number of deaths was 560,000 annually. In 2005, those figures were 1,372,900 and 570,280 respectively. The difference in these figures is statistically insignificant.

Moss and other critics point out that the war on cancer is not being won at all, but that statistics are being used in such a way as to give the appearance of advancements. For example, the ACS often cites improved survival rates as evidence of progress. They define the five-year survival rate as "living five years after diagnosis, whether disease-free, in remission, or under treatment with evidence of cancer." They report the five-year survival rate between 1974 and 1976 as 50 percent and the five-year survival rate between 1995 and 2000 as 64 percent. This appears promising until advancements in early detection are factored in. Because patients are being diagnosed at much earlier stages of cancer, they falsely appear to live longer.

Since the current state of cancer care today is far from perfect, satisfaction with the status quo seems an unlikely reason for lack of support and investigation of Essiac and other alternative therapies. If anything, the situation would warrant making changes and looking in other directions. Since that is not the case, other factors must be at play in the reluctance to consider the value of alternative therapies.

One factor in the lack of investigation into CAM modalities is the somewhat adversarial relationship that exists between allopathic and alternative medicine. Most practitioners of Western medicine simply do not acknowledge the validity of alternative medicine and therefore will do nothing to promote or advance its use. The minority of doctors who do support alternative therapies are often criticized and ostracized by their peers. This was evident during Rene Caisse's time, and it has continued into recent history.

One of the most notable cases of persecution involves Stanislaw R. Bursynski, MD, PhD, who was indicted on seventy-five counts of fraud for administering antineolplastons (his discovery) to cancer patients (Moss 2002). He suffered years of persecution (hearings, raids, and threats of prosecution) reminiscent of Rene Caisse, but with one exception. He had ample scientific data to support his work. But similar to Rene, his treatment involved a simple natural substance found in blood and urine. His defenders maintain that had his treatment been synthetic and patentable, he would have been immediately hailed as a hero for his valuable (and lucrative) discovery. Despite adversity, he runs the successful Bursynski Clinic in Houston, TX, where patients are offered his targeted therapy against cancer.

Another example of opposition to alternative medicine and the criticism of those MDs who break rank can be found on the website operated by Quackwatch, Inc., a non-profit corporation founded by retired psychiatrist Stephen Barrett, MD. Its purpose is to "combat health-related fraud, myths, fads, and fallacies" (Barrett 2006, para. 1). This seems an admirable mission, but close examination of the website reveals something interesting. The entire website is an indictment of all methods alternative. This is not to say that there are not perpetrators of fraud among those who claim to have alternative remedies. However, a patient going to this website will be warned against all forms of alternative medicine, including nutritional therapies, acupuncture, chiropractic, herbal, and Chinese medicine. According to Barrett, "Alternative medicine has become the politically correct term for questionable practices formerly labeled quack and fraudulent" (Quackwatch 2006, para. 1).

Further, his vitriol is not confined only to alternative therapies, but to institutions, proponents, and practitioners who advance it as well. For example, according to Quackwatch, the following physicians are "non-recommended" sources of health advice: Lorraine Day, MD, Bernie Seigel, MD, and Andrew Weil, MD, to name a few. In a section on cancer treatments, an extensive list of "dubious" treatments is posted, and among them is Essiac. The reason for its dubious distinction: "Several animal tests using samples of Essiac have shown no antitumor activity, nor did a review of data on eighty-six patients performed by the Canadian federal health department during the early 1980s" (Barrett and Herbert 2006, Essiac). This two-sentence appraisal demonstrates a "dubious" depth and quality of investigation, which is evident throughout the website. It is notable that no cautions are posted concerning any conventional medical treatments. This despite the fact that there were ninety-eight thousand preventable deaths from medical errors in 2004, representing the sixth leading cause of death in the United States that year (Wrong Diagnosis 2006).

In 2009, "Deaths from avoidable medical error more than doubled in the past decade, investigation shows. Preventable medical mistakes and infections are responsible for about 200,000 deaths in the United States each year, according to an investigation by the Hearst media corporation" (*Scientific American* 2009).

Another factor in the lack of clinical investigation of Essiac is a general reluctance of researchers to study natural substances in their entirety. An herb, for example, might contain hundreds of compounds, but researchers often try to isolate or focus on the compound they feel most responsible for eliciting a biological effect. The reasons for this are financially motivated. By most accounts, 80 percent of all conventional drugs are derived from, or conceived by, studying plants and herbs. But pharmaceutical companies routinely work to isolate an active ingredient, reproduce it synthetically, and patent it, with the goal of increasing profits.

Substances derived from the Madagascar periwinkle, the American mayapple, and the Pacific yew tree have been used in the creation of the cancer drugs Vincristine, Etoposide, and Paclitaxel, respectively. All of these synthetic drugs have toxic side effects. It is of interest that the components of Essiac tea in their natural plant form are all nontoxic. Yet, according to Moss, "The FDA has still not approved any non-toxic agents as treatments for cancer. NCI has still not conducted a single fair and competent study of any alternative cancer therapy" (2002, VIII).

So, despite the inadequacies of current cancer therapies, there is little impetus to change directions. There is also reluctance to change because the cancer industry is huge and entrenched, and it sustains the livelihoods of a large percentage of the population that provides and supports healthcare services. Although it may be tempting to assign malicious motives to those who profit from human suffering, that assessment would be unfair for the most part. As Moss put it, "The important point is that the suppression of unorthodox methods—and the promotion of the orthodox approach—takes place mainly at an objective, unconscious level. It is an outgrowth of underlying economic and social trends rather than of conscious design" (2002, 419).

In the current culture, treating disease is far more profitable than preventing it. With this in mind, it is an encouraging sign that the public is increasingly seeking out and using CAM therapies. Public perception and demand will be what dictates change.

# CONCLUSION

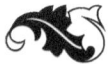

The herbal cancer remedy known as Essiac has stood the test of time. For nearly ninety years, it has been used by patients, most of who have been in advanced stages of cancer. Countless cases of easing of symptoms, remissions, and cures have been documented. It has received the endorsement of prominent physicians, and it has been the subject of petitions, appeals to governmental authorities, newspaper and magazine articles, radio talk shows, television documentaries, and a half dozen books. Its creator, Rene Caisse, RN, devoted most of her adult life to treating patients with the herbal remedy, most of whom had exhausted all conventional treatments. She spent most of her adult lifetime trying to have her vast clinical experience with cancer treatment recognized by the established medical community.

Despite this volume of evidence and huge public support, Rene and her supporters maintained that she had suffered persecution from the medical hierarchy that had placed impediments to having Essiac recognized as a legitimate form of treatment. Those who blocked the way countered that they could not approve Essiac without clinically testing the formula themselves. Rene steadfastly refused to divulge the formula until her years of clinical research were validated. Because of this stalemate, Essiac would never be officially recognized as a cancer drug in North America.

Demand for the herbal remedy continued despite its lack of official recognition. It would instead be marketed as an herbal tonic that anyone can purchase. It is manufactured by many different companies and goes by many different brand names. No medical claims can be made, but word of mouth and customer testimonials continue to abound.

A cursory investigation into Essiac is likely to yield only a condensed history and anecdotal evidence. Many "experts" claim that its value is totally unproven and that there has been no clinical research on it. However, a more thorough search will turn up numerous investigations into Essiac preparations and its component herbs. All of these have proven it to possess anti-cancer properties and to be safe and non-toxic. Further, the most intensive clinical studies conducted on an Essiac formulation took place in China over a three-year period. These studies yielded such positive data that the Chinese Ministry of Health issued the first-ever import permit for a non-traditional Chinese medicine for a Class A (life threatening) disease. Therefore, this same Essiac formulation is marketed as a cancer drug in China (where medical claims can be made), and as an herbal tonic in North America (where no medical claims can be made).

The state of cancer care today is far from perfect, with conventional cancer treatments such as chemotherapy and radiation having deleterious side effects and limited increases in survival time. Further, the cost of traditional care is skyrocketing. Because of this, many cancer sufferers are compelled to look elsewhere to improve their outcomes. However, Essiac has only minor possible side effects, and it has demonstrated an ability to alleviate the symptoms caused by traditional therapies. It has proven efficacy and non-toxicity, and it is priced affordably.

Mainstream doctors are most often reluctant to acknowledge the benefits of alternative therapies. Their dismissal or indifference is the result of many factors, but they can mainly be categorized as educational, social, and economic. However, the use of complementary/alternative medicine (CAM) by patients—including herbal therapies such as Essiac—has increased dramatically in the last twenty years, with or without their doctors' knowledge. CAM offers cancer sufferers an avenue of hope.

Every aspect of Essiac's history demonstrates a need for it to be investigated thoroughly and reliably in a clinical environment. It is far too often the last resort of those afflicted with cancer, and yet it continues to demonstrate favorable results. One can only wonder how well it would work if it were the first line of defense used to strengthen the immune system so that the body could eliminate the cancer cells on its own.

In Dr. Weil's words,
Ultimately, hopes for cures of cancer are equivalent to hopes for immune responses, because the immune

system has the potential to recognize and eliminate malignant tissue. The future of cancer treatment is not in bigger and better cytotoxic weapons (which will never be capable of killing malignant cells without also killing fast-growing normal cells). Instead, the future will bring immunotherapy capable of rousing a slumbering immune system to action. (1995, 269)

The dissatisfaction with current cancer care is driving patients to seek alternative care to augment (and sometimes replace) the standard care they receive. For this reason alone, Essiac and other alternative therapies should be carefully studied. In this way, patients can receive standardized quality treatments that benefit them and avoid harmful or worthless therapies.

In closing, the need for further clinical investigation of Essiac is warranted and crucial. Cancer is devastating to its victims and their loved ones, and it is epidemic in proportion. There is a vital need for therapies that boost the immune system and ameliorate suffering, and Essiac gives every indication of doing just that. It has proven efficacy and safety. It is a natural, inexpensive remedy, and its benefits need to be validated by traditional medicine so that cancer patients can more fully realize its potential.

# REFERENCES

American Cancer Society. "Statistics," American Cancer Society, 2006. Accessed March 20, 2006. http://www.cancer.org/docroot/STT/stt_0_2005asp?sitearea=STT&Level=1.

Balch, P. A., *Prescription for Herbal Healing: An Easy-to-Use A-Z Reference to Hundreds of Common Disorders and Their Herbal Remedies.* New York: Avery, 2002.

Barrett, S., "Quackwatch: A special message for cancer patients seeking 'alternative' treatments." Quackwatch (2006). Accessed March 22, 2006. http://www.quackwatch.org/01QuackeryRelatedTopics/altwary.html.

Barrett, S. and V. Herbert, "Questionable Cancer Therapies." Accessed March 22, 2006 from the World Wide Web. http://www.quackwatch.org/

Belkin, M. and D. B. Fitzgerald, "Tumor-damaging capacity of plant materials." *The Journal of the National Cancer Institute.* Aug *13*(1) (1952):139-55. Accessed February 10, 2006. http://www.ncbi.nih.gov/entrez/query.fcgi?cmd=Retrieve&db=pubmed&dopt=Abstract&list_uids=14946504&query_hl=1&tool=pubmed_docsum.

Berenson, A., "A cancer drug shows promise at a price that many can't pay." *The New York Times*, Feb. 15, 2006.

Boik, J., *Oregon Medical Press Online* (2003). Accessed September 8, 2005. http://www.ompress.com/community-faq-2.htm.

Boon, H., M. Stewart, M. A. Kennard, R. Gray, C. Sawka, and J. B. Brown, "Use of complementary/alternative medicine by breast cancer survivors in Ontario: prevalence and perceptions." *Journal of Clinical Oncology.* Jul. 18(13) (2000):2515-21. Accessed June 12, 2005.http://www.ncbi.nlm.nih.gov/entrez/query.fcgi?cmd=Retrieve&db=pubmed&dopt=Abstract&list_uids=10893281&query_hl=3&tool=pubmed_docsum.

Brinker, F., ND, *Herb Contraindications and Drug Interactions.* Sandy, Oregon: Eclectic Medical Publications, 1998.

Caisse, R. M., *I Was Canada's Cancer Nurse: The Story of ESSIAC.* New York: Maurine B. Cox, 1966. Diamond, S., "Science now confirms what the first nation's people have always known." *Flor-Essence* (2003).

Accessed February 9, 2006 http://floressencetea.com/ScienceNowconfirms.htm

Dombradi C. A. and S. Foldeak, "Screening report on the antitumor activity of purified arctium lappa extracts." *Tumori* May/Jun 52(3) (1966):173-5. Accessed January 30, 2006 http/www.ncbi.nlm.nih.gov/entrez/query.fcgi?CMD=search&DB=pubmed.

Douglass, W.C., "When the cure is worse than the sickness." *Real Health News*, Aug 30 (2002). Accessed October 3, 2005. http://www.aspartame.ca/page_c4.htm.

Duke, J. A., PhD, *The Green Pharmacy.* New York: St. Martin's Press, 1997.

Dy, G. K., L. Bekele, L. J. Hanson, A. Furth, S. Mandrekar, and J. A. Sloan, "Complementary and alternative medicine use by patients enrolled onto phase I clinical trials." *The Journal of Clinical Oncology.* Dec 1 22(23) (2004):4810-5. Accessed September 7, 2005. http://www.ncbi.nlm.nih.gov/entrez/query.fcgi?cmd=Retrieve&db=pubmed&dopt=Abstract&list_uids=15570083&query_hl=9&tool=pubmed_docsum.

Fong, J. K. F., MD, "Clinical summary on taking CESSIAC C-Formula and YUCCATIVE Y-Formula from 583 cases." *CESSIAC* (1996). Accessed September 8, 2005. http://www.cessiac.com/clincals/583%20cases.htm.

Genentech. Herceptin. "Phase III Clinical efficacy in first-line treatment & incidence and severity of cardiac dysfunction," (2005a). Accessed September 11, 2005.

http://www.gene.com/gene/common/inc/pi/her-ceptin.jsp?productSite=1.

Genentech. Avastin. Study 1 efficacy results, (2005b). Accessed September 15, 2006. http://www.gene.com/gene/products/information/oncology/avastin/insert.jsp

Glum, G. L., *Calling of an Angel.* Los Angeles, CA: Silent Walker Publishing, 1988.

Hanrahan, C., *Gale Encyclopedia of Alternative Medicine.* Gale Group, 2001. Accessed September 11, 2005. http://www.findarticles.com/p/articles/mi_g2603/is_0002/ai_2603000240.

Harmon, K., "Death from avoidable medical error more than doubles in past decade, investigation shows." *Scientific American*, Aug 10, 2009.

Harrar, S. N., "Beating Breast Cancer." *Prevention* (2006): 42.

Harris P., I. G. Finlay, A. Cook, K. J. Thomas, and K. Hood, "Complementary and alternative medicine use by patients with cancer in Wales: a cross sectional survey." *Complementary Therapeutic Medicine*, Dec 11(4) (2003):249-53. Accessed September 7, 2005. http://www.ncbi.nlm.nih.gov/entrez/query.fcgi?cmd=Retrieve&db=pubmed&dopt=Abstract&list_uids=15022659&query_hl=5&tool=pubmed_docsum.

Ivey, D. M. *Clinic of Hope.* Toronto: Dundurn Press, 2004.

Kaegi, E. MB, ChB, MSc, Unconventional therapies for cancer: 1. Essiac. The Task Force on Alternative

Therapies of the Canadian Breast Cancer Research Initiative, 1998. *Canadian Medical Association Journal.* April 7, 1998; *158*:897-902

Lengacher, C. A., M. P. Bennett, K. E. Kip, R. Keller, M. S. LaVance, and L. S. Smith, "Frequency of use of complementary and alternative medicine in women with breast cancer." *Oncology Nurse Forum.* Nov-Dec 29(10) (2002):1445-52. Accessed September 7, 2005. http://www.ncbi.nlm.nih.gov/entrez/query.fcgi?cmd=Retrieve&db=pubmed&dopt=Abstract&list_uids=12432415&query_hl=1&tool=pubmed_docsum.

Leonard S. S., D. Keil, T. Mehlman, S. Proper, X. Shi, and G. K. Harris, "Essiac tea: scavenging of reactive oxygen species and effects of DNA damage." *Journal of Ethnopharmacology.* Jan 16:103(2) (2006):288-96. Accessed February 7, 2006.http://www.ncbi.nlm.nih.gov/entrez/query.fcgi?cmd=Retrieve&db=pubmed&dopt=Abstract&list_uids=16226859&tool=iconfft&query_hl=5&tool=pubmed_docsum.

Lin C. C., J. M. Lu, J. J. Yang, S. C. Chuang, and T. Ujiie, "Anti-inflammatory and radical scavenge effects of arctium lappa." *American Journal of Chinese Medicine.* 24(2) (1996):127-37. Accessed September 27, 2005.http://www.ncbi.nlm.nih.gov/entrez/query.fcgi?cmd=Retrieve&db=PubMed&list_uids=8874669&query_hl=13&tool=pubmed_d.

Lui, Mr. and Ms. Chan, "C" Formula acute toxicity test. Guangdong Provincial Institute of Materia Medica,

Pharmacology Department, (1995a). Accessed September 8, 2005. http://www.cessiac.com/clinicals/C toxic test.htm

Lui, Mr. and Ms. Chan, "Y" Formula acute toxicity test. Guangdong Provincial Institute of Materia Medica, Pharmacology Department, (1995b). Accessed September 8, 2005. http://www.cessiac.com / clinicals/Y toxic test.htm.

Lui, Mr. and Ms. Chan, "Y" Formula acute toxicity test. Guangdong Provincial Institute of Materia Medica, Pharmacology Department, (1995c). Accessed September 8, 2005. http://www.cessiac.com /clinicals/tumor inhibition.htm.

MedlinePlus. "Drug Information: Paclitaxel. A service of the US National Library of Science & the National Institutes of Health," (2003a). Accessed February 10, 2006. http://www.nlm.nih.gov/medlineplus/druginfo/medmaster/a698035.html

MedlinePlus. "Drug Information: Decadron. A service of the US National Library of Science & the National Institutes of Health," (2003b). Accessed February 10, 2006.http://www.nlm.nih.gov/medlineplus/druginfo/medmaster/a682792.html.

MedlinePlus. "Drug Information: Herceptin. A service of the US National Library of Science & the National Institutes of Health," (2003c). Accessed February 13, 2006. http://www.nlm.nih.gov/medlineplus/druginfo/medmaster/a699019.html

MedlinePlus. "Drug Information: Avastin. A service of the US National Library of Science & the National Institutes of Health," (2005d). Accessed February 15, 2006. http://www.nlm.nih.gov/medlineplus/druginfo/uspdi/500579.html.

MedlinePlus. "Herbs and supplements: Essiac. A service of the US National Library of Science & the National Institutes of Health," (2005e). Accessed February 23, 2006. http//www.nlm.nih.gov/medlineplus/druginfo/natural.patient-essiac.html.

Morita K., T. Kada, and M. Namiki, "A desmutagenic factor isolated from burdock (arctium lappa linne.). *Mutat Res.*" Oct. *129*(1) (1984):25-31 Accessed September 27, 2005. http://www.ncbi.nlm.nih.gov/entrez/query.fcgi?cmd=Retrieve&db=pubmed&dopt+Abstract&list_uids=63874668query_ hl=10&tool=pubmed_docsum.

Moss, R. W., PhD, *The Cancer Industry.* State College, PA: Equinox Press, 2002.

Moss, R. PhD, *Herbs Against Cancer.* Lemont, PA: Equinox Press, 2005.

National Cancer Institute, US National Institutes of Health. (2005). "Essiac/Flor-Essence human/clinical studies." Accessed January 27, 2006.http://www.cancer.gov/cancertopics/pdq/cam/essiac/HealthProfessional/page5.

Olson, C., *ESSIAC: A Native Herbal Cancer Remedy.* Pagosa Springs, CA: Kali Press, 1998.

Ottenweller, J., K. Putt, E. J. Blumenthal, S. Dhawale, and S.W. Dhawale, "Inhibition of prostate cancer-cell proliferation by Essiac." *The Journal of Alternative and Complementary Medicine.* Aug. 10(4) (2004):687-91. Accessed May 19, 2005. http://www.ncbi.nlm.nih.gov/entrez/query.fcgi?cmd=Retrieve&db=pubmed&dopt=Abstract&list_uids=15353028&tool=iconabstr&query_hl =6&tool=pubmed_docsum.

Percival, J., *The Essiac Handbook.* Monbahus, France: Bernard Barbieux Associates, 1994.

Quillin, P., PhD, RD, CNS, *Beating Cancer with Nutrition.* Carlsbad, CA: Nutrition Times Press, Inc., 2005.

Research Section of Pharmacology, Institute of Materia Medica of Guangdong Province. A study on the tumor-inhibition effect of combined use of "C" Formula and "Y" Formula, 1995. Accessed September 8, 2005. http://www.cessiac.com/clinicals/tumor%20inhibition.htm.

Richardson, MA, Dr. P. H., T. Sanders, MPH, C. Tamayo, MD, C. Perez, MPH, and J. L. Palmer, PhD, "Flor-Essence® herbal tonic use in North America: a profile of general consumers and cancer patients." Centers for Alternative Medicine Research and Health Promotion Research and Development, The University of Texas-Houston School of Public Health, Foresight Link Corporation, Ontario, Canada & the Department of Biostatistics, The University of Texas MD Anderson Cancer Center, 2000. Accessed September 9, 2005.

http://www.floressencetea.com/HGherbalgram.html.

Richardson, M. A., L. C. Masse, K. Nanny, and C. Sanders, "Discrepant views of oncologists and cancer patients on complementary/alternative medicine." *Supportive Care in Cancer.* Nov 12(11) (2004):797-804. Accessed September 7, 2005. http://www.ncbi.nlm.nih.gov/entrez/query.fcgi?cmd=Retrieve&db=pubmed&dopt=Abstract&list.

Snow, S. and M. Klein, *Essiac Essentials: The Remarkable Herbal Cancer Fighter.* New York: Kensington Publishing Corp, 1999.

Snow, Sheila and Mali Klein, *Essiac: The Secrets of Rene Caisse's Herbal Pharmacy.* Dublin: Newleaf, 2001.

Sparber, A., L. Bauer, G. Curt, D. Eisenberg, T. Levin, and S. Parks, "Use of complementary and alternative medicine by adult patients participating in cancer clinical trials." *Oncology Nurses Forum* Jul 27(6) (2000):887-8. Accessed September 7, 2005. http://www.ncbi.nlm.nih.gov/entrez/query.fcgi?cmd=Retrieve&db=pubmed&dopt=Abstract&list_uids=10833691&query_hl=10&tool=pubmed_docsum.

Tai, J., S. Cheung, S. Wong, and C. Lowe, "In vitro comparison of Essiac and Flor-Essence on human tumor cell lines." *Oncology Reports.* Feb. 11(2) (2004): 471-6.

Tamayo, C., M. A. Richardson, S. Diamond, and I. Skoda, "The chemistry and biological activity of herbs used in Flor-Essence herbal tonic and Essiac." *Phytotherapy Research.* Feb 14(1) (2000):1-14.

Thomas, R., *The Essiac Report.* Third edition. Los Angeles, CA: The Alternative Treatment Information Network, 1993.

Tierra, Dr. M., *Treating Cancer with Herbs: An Integrative Approach.* Twin Lakes, WI: Lotus Press, 2003.

Vaughan, Z., *I Beat Cancer.* Oxnard, CA: Awareness Publishing, 2003.

Weil, A., MD., *Spontaneous Healing.* New York: Random House, 1995.

"Death from medical misadventure: patient safety in Hospitals." Healthgrades, 2004. Accessed March 22, 2006. http://www.wrongdiagnosis.com/m/medical_misadventure/deaths.htm.

Yan, R., Q. Lao, and Z. Chen, Clinical report on the therapeutic effect of "C" Formula& "Y" Formula from 39 cases. The Institute of Pharmaceutical Research of Guangdong Province. Accessed September 12, 2005. http://www.cessiac.com/clinicals/39%20Cases.h

www.ingramcontent.com/pod-product-compliance
Lightning Source LLC
Chambersburg PA
CBHW051428280526
45785CB00003B/1209